LECTURE NOTES ON DERMATOLOGY

LECTURE NOTES ON
Dermatology

BETHEL SOLOMONS
M.A. M.D. F.R.C.P.I.

*Consultant Dermatologist to Chelmsford and
Essex General Hospital, Herts and
Essex General Hospital*

FOURTH EDITION

BLACKWELL SCIENTIFIC PUBLICATIONS

OXFORD LONDON EDINBURGH MELBOURNE

© 1965, 1969, 1973, 1977 by Blackwell Scientific Publications
Osney Mead, Oxford, England
8 John Street, London WC1, England
9 Forrest Road, Edinburgh, Scotland
P.O. Box 9, North Balwyn, Victoria, Australia

First published 1965
Reprinted 1966
Second edition 1969
Third edition 1973
Reprinted 1975
Fourth edition 1977

Solomons, Bethel
Lecture notes on dermatology.—4th ed.
1. Dermatology
I. Title
616.5   RL71
ISBN 0-632-00145-3

Distributed in the U.S.A. by
J. B. Lippincott Company, Philadelphia,
and in Canada by
J. B. Lippincott Company of
Canada Ltd, Toronto

Printed and bound in Great Britain by
the Alden Press, Oxford

Contents

CONTENTS

Preface to Fourth Edition

A great amount of this revised edition consists of new material, especially in regard to recent innovations in treatment and the re-orientating of old concepts in relation to aetiology. The importance of immunological mechanisms is introduced as far as is pertinent. Many outmoded remedies have been discarded.

Dr W.H.Jopling has revised the section he wrote on leprosy, and Dr J.K.Oates has made alterations to his account of syphilis and Reiter's disease, whilst adding a description of chronic gonococcal dermatitis, and to both of them I am very grateful. I also wish to thank Richard Solomons for his good advice, and Miss Gwen Smart for retyping the book.

The essential aim of the book remains the same, i.e. as an introduction to dermatology for students, and an early reference for general practitioners.

Finally, as always, I am indebted to the patience and cooperation of the publishers.

37 Devonshire Place   BETHEL SOLOMONS
London W1N 1PE

CHAPTER 1

Anatomy, Physiology and Pathology

ANATOMY AND PHYSIOLOGY

Apart from its apparent function as an elastic envelope to walk about in, the skin has several other important qualities. It is waterproof and airtight, although some substances may be absorbed by it.

It acts as a form of thermostat, the heat of the body being regulated by the blood vessels and by sweating.

It protects underlying organs from physical, chemical and other injuries.

It acts as a relay station between external influences and internal organs by means of its tremendously complicated network of nerve terminals.

It acts as an organ of expression, betraying the innermost feelings of anxiety by sweating, fear by pallor, and anger by redness.

It is an important store for water, containing 18–20 per cent of the total water content of the body, and this amount decreases with age. It is mainly distributed in the dermis.

Histology

The skin is divided into three principal layers:

1. the epidermis;
2. the dermis;
3. the subcutaneous tissue.

Epidermis

The *epidermis* is subdivided into four layers: (a) the basal layer or stratum germinativum, (b) the malpighian or prickle cell layer or stratum spinosum, (c) the granular layer or stratum granulosum, (d) the horny layer or stratum corneum (Fig. 1). (An extra layer, the so-called lucid layer, lies above the granular layer, and is found only on the palms and soles.) The cells in the basal layer gradually evolve into the cells of the horny layer at random, and make their way to the horny surface, changing only in shape and size, as they pass through the malpighian and granular layer.

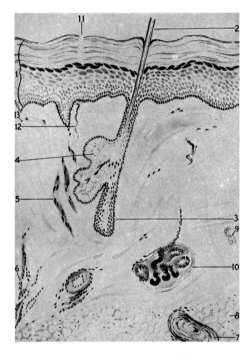

FIG. 1. Diagram of constituents of the skin.

1. Epidermis. 2. Hair. 3. Hair follicle. 4. Sebaceous gland. 5. Muscle fibres of M. arrector pili. 6. Blood vessel. 7. Pacinian body. 8. Fat lobules. 9. Cutaneous nerve. 10. Sweat glands. 11. Sweat duct opening. 12. Terminal nerve fibrils. 13. Collagen bundles.

The *basal layer* lies deepest in the epidermis, and next to the dermis. It consists of two types of cell:

(i) basal cells;
(ii) melanocytes.

Basal cells are columnar in shape, their long axis being at right angles to the dermis beneath them. They contain a dark staining oval or elongated nucleus which lies in deeply basophilic cytoplasm. They are joined to each other by intercellular bridges.

Melanocytes are dendritic cells in which melanin is formed. Melanocytes all arise from the neural crest. Epidermal melanocytes appear as a haphazard horizontal arrangement above the dermal junction.

The *malpighian layer* is also called the prickle cell layer, because the cells appear to be held together by prickles; they are actually intercellular bridges, which provide greater stability to the polygonal prickle cells.

The *granular layer* is composed of one to four rows of diamond-shaped cells, filled with deeply basophilic granules.

The *horny layer* normally contains no nuclei and is continuously shed from the surface. Only by means of the electron microscope can intercellular spaces be seen. Its hardness is due to keratin (see p. 8).

The epidermis also possesses the following appendages:

1. the eccrine glands;
2. the apocrine glands;
3. the sebaceous glands;
4. the hair;
5. the nails.

THE SWEAT GLANDS
There are two varieties in man, the eccrine and the apocrine. They regulate heat, causing heat loss by evaporation; and they improve the grip. They arise as downgrowths from the epidermis.

THE ECCRINE GLANDS
These exist all over the skin, but not in mucous membranes, the total number varying between 2 and 5 million; the numbers vary greatly according to the site. There are obviously, a lot more on the palms than the legs. The gland starts as a coil in the dermis, and opens

invisibly on the skin surface. The secretion is a clear watery fluid, 99–99·5 per cent water, also containing chlorides, lactic acid, urea, nitrogen and other substances.

THE APOCRINE GLANDS

These are large sweat glands, whose ducts open into hair follicles to which they are attached, and rarely on to the surface of the skin. They are coiled tubular glands, with a duct leading down to a coil of secretory tubules. They are found in the axillae, ano-genital areas, nipple and areola, but do not develop fully until puberty. Modified apocrine glands occur in the external ear, producing wax; and on the eyelids, where cystic blockage may occur. The product of the glands is a whitish, sterile fluid, containing proteins, carbohydrates and other substances. It is evoked in response to stress, pain, fright or sexual activity.

THE SEBACEOUS GLANDS

These are found all over the body, except on the palms, soles and dorsa of the feet. They are most numerous on the scalp, face, fore-head, and chin. The glands have no lumen and their secretion is the result of decomposition of their cells, most of it being discharged through the sebaceous duct into a pilo-sebaceous follicle. They are multi-lobulated, and appear as a pouch hanging on the outer side of the follicle. The secretion is known as sebum, and contains fatty acids, cholesterol and other substances. The exact function of sebum is still in dispute.

THE HAIR

A hair consists of a root containing non-keratinized cells, and a shaft composed of keratinized cells. The shaft extends from the skin surface to the free end of the hair. The root and its lower end are called the hair-bulb and contain the hair matrix cells. They comprise all the part below the skin surface, and lie in what is called the hair-follicle. A pointed projection of the dermis protrudes into the hair-bulb, and this is the papilla. It is luxuriantly supplied with nerves and blood vessels, and contains melanin which is responsible for the pigment of dark hair.

The distribution of the hair is universal except for the palms, soles, dorsal aspect of the distal phalanges of the hands and feet, the penis, the labia minora and the lips.

There are three types of hair:

1. downy or lanugo hairs which cover the face (except the beard and moustache areas), hands and limbs;

2. long soft hairs, which cover the scalp, beard, moustache, axillae, and pubes;

3. stiff hairs which are found on the eyebrows, eyelids, and in the nose and auditory meatus.

Hair growth varies according to the area. The average daily rate of scalp hair growth is 0·37 mm, and a hair may continue growing for from 2 to 6 years before falling. An average number of scalp hairs is 100,000, and the usual daily loss is 20 to 100. This is comforting consolation for those who imagine they are going to lose all their hair when they find a daily number on their brush or comb.

The reason why baldness does not occur as a result of this constant fall is due to the cyclical growth of hair. In every single hair follicle there is a resting period followed by a growth period; the loss of hair is not noticeable because neighbouring follicles have differently-timed cycles, and are at the same time at different phases of the cycle. These phases are known as the anagen phase (the active growing phase), the resting or telogen phase, and the intermediate or catagen phase.

On other areas such as the trunk, eyebrows and limbs the growing period of the hairs lasts about 6 months, so that the hairs do not grow to a great length.

The influences on hair growth are complex and perplexing. The male hormone testosterone maintains the sex hairs of men and women. It also provokes the growth of beard hair, yet its presence is a condition for the development of male scalp baldness. Eunuchs never become bald. Other hormones have little effect on hair growth except for the pituitary which, through its connection with the adrenals and the gonads has an indirect influence.

The function of the hair is to protect the skin against minor harmful influences; for example, eyebrows direct sweat away from the eyes, and the nasal vibrissae filter air. It also acts as a thermoregulator, a promoter of sweat evaporation, is a sensitive tactile organ, and provides sexual attraction.

The health of the hair depends on the health of the individual. The visible hair is a dead structure, and no amount of singeing, brushing or oiling will alter its fundamental vitality, although its appearance may be improved.

NAILS

Nails are translucent, compact, solid plates of keratin. The matrix lies beneath the nail-fold. The paronychium is the soft tissue surrounding the nail border.

The average *growth rate* is 0·1 mm daily. A finger nail takes about 100–150 days to reproduce itself, and a toe nail about three times as long. Growth may be affected by disease, and nail shedding, splitting or ridging may accompany long illnesses, or malnutrition. In some cases, there is no obvious cause for such nail disorders. Nail-growth is increased by nail-biting and, like hair, their growth is accelerated in summer-time.

Their *function* is the indispensable one of picking up small objects. They are also bright ornaments to the fingers, and in disease may often be indicators of internally situated disorders.

Dermis

The dermis may be divided into two parts:

    1. the papillary;
    2. the reticular.

The *papillary part* lies snugly against the epidermis above. The papillae strike up into it at irregular intervals, so that the alternating areas of epidermis which drop down produce the effect of a draped curtain. These epidermal drapes are called rete pegs.

Most of the papillae contain blood vessels, and some contain nerve elements, such as tactile corpuscles.

The *reticular part* contains connective tissue bundles, below which lies the subcutaneous tissue.

The dermis contains the following structures:

    (a) connective tissue fibres;
    (b) cellular elements;
    (c) blood vessels;
    (d) nerves;
    (e) muscles;
    (f) lymphatcis.

CONNECTIVE TISSUE FIBRES

There are three varieties: collagenous, elastic and reticulin.

Collagen fibres form 75 per cent of the total. Collagen is an albuminoid substance of which the bundles are comprised. These present a wavy appearance, and are held together by a ground substance. Fibroblasts lie between the bundles.

Elastic fibres run parallel or obliquely to the collagen, and enclose the bundles.

Reticulin fibres are composed of collagen fibrils, and probably ensure stability between dermis and epidermis.

CELLULAR ELEMENTS

A. *In health*

1. Migratory cells

    (a) Leucocytes lie sparsely around blood vessels and lymphatics.

    (b) Histiocytes resemble fibroblasts, having large round or oval kidney-shaped nuclei. They are also called reticulin cells. Their function is to absorb specific material, and form reticulin fibres. Under certain conditions they may change into epithelioid cells (see below).

2. Fixed cells

    (a) fibroblasts are spindle-shaped with elongated nuclei.

    (b) mast cells are histiocytic and spindle-shaped with an oval or round nucleus. They produce heparin and histamine. Normal skin contains few of them.

B. *In disease*

Apart from polymorphonuclear leucocytes, and lymphocytes, which play their accustomed roles in inflammatory disease, other cells sometimes play a diagnostic part in skin disorders.

Eosinophils are significant in dermatitis herpetiformis.

Macrophages are phagocytizing histiocytes, and when fused, appear as multi-nucleated foreign body giant cells. As such, they particularly appear in gout.

Epithelioid cells are altered histiocytes and together may form Langhans giant cells, and as such appear in tuberculous, sarcoidal and syphilitic lesions.

Plasma cells occur in most chronic inflammatory conditions. The functions of the plasma cell are the synthesis of antibodies and gamma globulin.

Foam cells are histiocytes ingesting lipoids, and are easily identified in the lesions of xanthoma.

BLOOD VESSELS

The blood supply nourishes the skin and removes its waste products, as well as playing an important role in the regulation of body temperature.

A capillary plexus exists between the dermis and the subcutaneous tissue, and in the sub-papillary area. Always varying, its position can never be accurately defined. The deep vessels have three layers of cells, the superficial vessels have one.

The glomus consists of an arterial segment, the Sucquet-Hoyer canal, and a venous segment, and is found on the tips of the fingers, toes, under the nails, also in the palms, soles, in the ears and centre of the face. It is a local temperature regulator.

NERVES

The skin is supplied from non-medullated and medullated fibres, which reach it from bundles in the subcutaneous tissue.

The sensations of touch, spatial discrimination, and temperature on hairless skin such as the palms, soles, lips, nipples, penis and clitoris, have until recently been thought of as being mediated by specialized end-organs, named Meissner's tactile bodies, Pacinian corpuscles, Krause's end bulbs, or Merkel-Ranvier discs. This conception is now in doubt, and such sensations are considered nowadays to be mediated through the free sensory nerve endings in the epidermis.

MUSCLES

Smooth or involuntary muscle is found all over the skin, except on the neck, and in the facial muscles of expression. Smooth muscle is attached to the hair follicles, as arrectores pilorum which on contraction produce 'gooseflesh', the tunica dartos of the scrotum, and the fibres of the areola of the nipple.

LYMPHATIC VESSELS

Few exist, and in the dermis present a spongy network, passing to deeper and larger plexuses in the subcutaneous tissue.

SKIN SURFACE LIPIDS

These cover the surface with a watery greasy film, called sebum, whose function is debatable.

Their production varies in different areas, and individuals. These lipids increase as adolescence approaches, and declines with advancing age, the levels in males being higher than in females. Hypersecretion, or abnormal sebum composition seems to be involved in the aetiology of acne, although its role is far from clear.

KERATIN

This is a fibrous protein, found in the horny layer of the epidermis, hair and nails. It is resistant to digestion by trypsin and pepsin, and is insoluble in water, dilute acids, alkalis and organic solvents.

WATER

The skin contains 18–20 per cent of the total water-content of the body. There is continuous invisible evaporation from the surface.

PIGMENTATION

The colour of normal skin originates from:

1. melanin;
2. oxyhaemoglobin;
3. reduced haemoglobin;
4. carotene.

Melanin results from the enzymatic oxidation of tyrosine by tyrosinase, and during the reaction dopa acts as a catalyst.

Tyrosinase

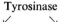

Tyrosin (precursor)→Dopa→(Intermediates)→Melanin
(dihydroxyphenylalanine)

Both melanogenesis and melanin pigmentation are also influenced by genetic and hormonal factors.

ABSORPTION

This occurs to a considerable degree, and the skin's absorptive capacity is greatly increased by abrasion. Hormones can be rubbed in, and it has been shown that iodine sprayed on the skin may be detected in the urine 20 minutes later. It has also been proved that water may be absorbed.

SENSATION

There are four types of sensation: pain, touch, cold and warmth, which are distinguished objectively and subjectively.

1. Pain sense. Pain may be caused by physical, chemical or mechanical irritation.

2. Touch sense. Touch spots are irregularly placed and are more concentrated where discrimination is acute. Touch stimuli are received from hair follicles, and the intervening skin.

3. Itching sense. This arises from terminal nerve-endings close to the skin surface (itching does not occur when the epidermis is absent).

4. Temperature sense. This sense is probably mediated through the free sensory nerve endings in the epidermis.

PATHOLOGY

The pathological changes found in skin diseases are often not diagnostic. The pathologist has to rely to a great extent on the clinical information supplied to him, which frequently is too trivial to be of much assistance. It should be a cardinal rule that a good description of the case be sent with the specimen. Even so, in many cases, the pathologist may only state that the findings are compatible with the clinical ones, such is the close histological resemblance of certain skin diseases. In some conditions, however, his report reveals or confirms the diagnosis.

The terminology of the dermatological pathologist contains some words peculiar to the specialty, and others which are used generally in pathology. It is essential to know some of the former, so that the more obvious minutiae of histological sections may be understood.

The following are the commonest changes in the epidermis:

1. Hyperkeratosis, which is hypertrophy of the horny layer. This is most classically seen in a corn.

2. Parakeratosis is the retention of nuclei in the cells of the horny layer. It is well seen in psoriasis, and other scaly conditions.

3. Acanthosis is an increase in the depth of the prickle-cell layer. It occurs in psoriasis, warts, and other conditions.

4. Spongiosis is inter-cellular oedema, a part of the picture of dermatitis and eczema.

5. Acantholysis is a detachment of epidermal cells from each other, which produces clefts, vesicles and bullae in the epidermis. It occurs in the bullous condition called pemphigus.

The following are the commonest changes in the dermis.

1. Hypertrophy or atrophy of fibrous tissue, as in a keloid, or senile skin, respectively.

2. Capillary changes, as in lupus erythematosus, or scleroderma.

3. Collagen degeneration, as in senile skin, or scleroderma.

Immunology

The role that immunological processes play in skin diseases is as yet poorly defined. Many suggestions related to such processes are tentative. It has, however, been inferred by many investigators that such relationships exist in lupus erythematosus, systemic sclerosis, pemphigus, the early stages of sarcoidosis, in the erythema nodosum of leprosy, and perhaps in dermatitis herpetiformis.

Investigators' nets have been widely cast in other directions too; they have peripherally covered contact dermatitis, urticaria and atopic eczema, for example, diseases whose basic mechanisms are poorly understood. Investigations may yet show that immunology is a very important aspect of skin diseases, and more importantly provides clues to more effective prophylactic and/or curative treatment for the unfortunate patient.

Allergy is an unusual or increased reaction following an initial exposure to any external agent, physical, chemical or biological, which is commonly harmless to most individuals. Most allergic reactions have their basis in an immunological reaction, i.e. an interaction between antigen and antibody. The commonest skin conditions reflecting an allergic state are urticaria, atopic eczema and contact dermatitis, and are dealt with elsewhere.

For detailed consideration of immunological reactions see an immunological textbook.

CHAPTER 2

History, Examination and Diagnosis

The traditional approach to a patient with a skin disease has usually, in the past, been a matter of observation. That is to say, examination and description of the lesion preceded any investigation into the history of the patient's condition. Almost all skin diseases can be diagnosed in this manner, because the signs necessary to make a diagnosis are immediately visible. Too often this method causes one to abbreviate history taking, a course which has many pitfalls. It minimizes the doctor–patient relationship from the start, when good rapport between them is often essential to effective treatment.

The recognition of the various types of lesion which may occur is the first essential towards making a diagnosis, a task sometimes more difficult than it sounds. But before this is done the patient should be put at ease, and of course all the senses must meanwhile be allert to pick up clues to the diagnosis as the patient approaches the doctor, just as in the diagnosis of a disorder of any other system. The author, in fact, believes that a personal approach is more rewarding than the impersonal one. The patient who has pruritus ani, or a sub-mammary rash, or lesions elsewhere on a clothed area, be it chest, abdomen, back or groin, should be questioned generally, so that an idea of the evolution and the symptomatology of the disease can be acquired. The patient will also be more co-operative and relaxed, and subsequently his equanimity will be maintained when submitted, naked, if necessary, to the analytical gaze of the physician.

While bearing in mind the importance of the doctor–patient relationship it is not a necessity in, for example, the removal of warts.

Whichever method is applied, the skin disease must not be treated separately from the patient, for treating the part will never cure the whole.

In skin disease, as in diseases of any other system, it is essential to keep an open mind about the diagnosis during the history and examination. In a weak moment, one may be unintentionally misguided by a doctor's letter accompanying the patient, or by the patient's idea of the diagnosis. Sometimes the dermatologist may be confronted by a patient who speaks of his troublesome wart, and this statement may be confirmed by his doctor, who owing to a cursory examination, or bad light, has failed to note that the lesion is a corn. The wrong treatment for this condition, as for many others, can lead to unnecessary complications, and delay in healing.

The diagnosis of any disease is an exciting exercise in the use of deductive powers, not least where skin diseases are concerned.

A working classification of common disorders, a knowledge of gross lesions and their distribution, combined with constructive history taking, should result in the correct diagnosis in all but uncommon diseases. For the latter, wide experience and supplementary aids, both histological and biochemical, will be required to discover the answer.

History Taking

A good history is often essential, particularly in chronic cases. This includes name, address, age, marital state, number of children, and occupation. Some of these factors may give a preliminary clue.

The following questions should be asked, although many may be excluded, if one is confident about the diagnosis, either as a result of some pointed answers as the patient is being questioned, or because one has seen and recognized the lesions. A complete history should include the following questions, but, as has been said, many will be irrelevant in some cases, and with experience, the pertinent ones to ask will be obvious.

PRESENT COMPLAINT

> Where did it start?
> Did it spread?
> Does it come and go?
> Is it wet, or dry?
> Does it itch?

TIME OF ONSET

The following questions are neither inclusive nor exclusive.

Were you subject to:

Infancy:	atopic dermatitis or infantile eczema
	naevi
	pyogenic infections
Childhood:	warts
	ringworm
	urticaria
	alopecia areata
Adolescence:	acne
Middle age:	neurodermatoses and tumours
Old age:	tumours, benign and malignant?

PERSONAL HISTORY

How does the patient sleep? Insomnia is usually a reflection of tension.

Do any foods or liquids make the rash worse? Chocolate sometimes aggravates acne; alcohol, hot liquids and coffee and tea may make rosacea worse.

Are the periods regular, and does their occurrence upset the rash? Both factors may influence acne and rosacea.

What cosmetics does the patient use?

What hobbies has the patient? The answer may reveal a cause of contact dermatitis.

What is the patient's job?

Has the rash any relationship to seasons? Acne, psoriasis and ichthyosis are less troublesome in summer, pityriasis rosea is more common in autumn and winter, and plant dermatitis in spring and summer.

FAMILY HISTORY

This is important when any of the conditions in chapter 20 are being considered, besides alopecia, atopic eczema, psoriasis, rosacea, seborrhoeic dermatitis, and urticaria.

When infective conditions such as impetigo, pediculosis, or scabies are present, contacts must be ascertained.

The next hurdle is *the identification of lesions*. One of the most important factors for this examination is good light. Many misdiagnoses are made because either the patient casts his shadow on the rash or the light is not powerful enough. Facilities must exist for complete examination of the patient if necessary.

The lesions of skin diseases may be primary or secondary.

PRIMARY LESIONS ARE

Macules
These are flat, circumscribed, discoloured lesions, of varying shapes and sizes, not raised above the skin.

Papules
These are raised, firm circumscribed lesions up to a centimetre in size.

Weals
This is a circumscribed type of elevation associated with itching or tingling.

Nodules
These have the same characteristics as papules but are larger, and usually can be felt to lie more deeply in the skin.

Tumours
These are larger than nodules, and may be elevated or very deeply placed in the skin.

Vesicles
These are well-defined small collections of fluid.

Bullae
These are large vesicles.

Pustules
These are circumscribed elevations of free purulent fluid. In some diseases, pustules may be sterile, as in acne.

SECONDARY LESIONS

Scales
These are dry or greasy masses of dead tissue from the horny layer depending on the condition. In psoriasis they may be dry and silvery and in seborrhoeic dermatitis, greasy and yellowish.

Crusts
Crusts must be carefully differentiated from scales, and the novice often confuses them. Crusts are masses of dried exudate, bacteria and leucocytes. They are a dirty yellow colour, and may be soft, dry and friable, or thick and hard. The surface of a crust is more uneven than that of a scale. They are not composed of well-defined layers, as scales are, and their general consistency is more lumpy.

Ulcers
These are irregularly-shaped excavations, resulting from necrosis of tissue including complete loss of epidermis and dermis. Each ulcer must be described in terms of shape, floor, base, edge and secretion. All ulcers leave a scar when they heal.

Scars
Scars are the result of damage to the dermis.
    Two peculiarities associated with secondary lesions need to be described. They are:

    1. Koebner's phenomenon.
    2. Nikolsky's sign.

Koebner's phenomenon is the appearance in a patient, usually with psoriasis or lichen planus, of features of these diseases in an area of skin that has been traumatized. For example, a patient with psoriasis is scratched by a thorn or nail; within a short time, psoriasis may appear in the injured area. These are the commonest conditions giving rise to this phenomenon, although plane warts may occasionally do so.
Nikolsky's sign is a sign elicited in pemphigus and describes the facility with which an apparently normal epidermis can be separated from the dermis by pinching or rubbing it.

A summary of the different types of lesions and some of the conditions associated with them

1. Nature

MACULES

Measles
Freckles
Naevus flammeus
Drug eruptions

Neurofibromatosis (café-au-lait spots)
Vitiligo
Addison's disease

SCALY MACULES

Tinea corporis
Pityriasis rosea

Seborrhoeic dermatitis
Pityriasis versicolor

PAPULES

Acne
Warts
Pigmented naevi
Xanthomata
Granuloma pyogenicum

Melanoma
Basal-cell carcinoma (rodent ulcer)
Molluscum contagiosum
Tuberculids

SCALY PAPULES

Psoriasis
Lichen planus
Atopic dermatitis

Contact dermatitis
Localized neurodermatitis
Syphilis

WEALS

Urticaria

Insect bites

NODULES

Warts
Haemangiomata
Chilblains
Erythema nodosum
Erythema induratum
Molluscum contagiosum

Kerato-acanthoma
Syphilis
Basal cell carcinoma
Lipomata
Neurofibromata

VESICLES

Herpes zoster
Herpes simplex
Insect bites
Chicken-pox
Contact dermatitis

Burns
Atopic dermatitis
Dermatitis herpetiformis
Scabies

BULLAE

Erythema multiforme
Pemphigus
Pemphigoid
Dermatitis herpetiformis
Impetigo

Herpes zoster
Contact dermatitis (poison ivy)
Insect bites
Drug eruptions (sulphonamides, barbiturates)

PUSTULES

Folliculitis
Acne
Rosacea
Chicken-pox

Herpes zoster
Herpes simplex
Smallpox

CRUSTS

Any vesicular or
  bullous dermatitis

Any ulcerating disease

SCARS

Any ulcerating disease

ULCERS

Trauma
Self-inflicted conditions;
  e.g. dermatitis artefacta
Bedsores
Venous stasis

Basal cell carcinoma
Squamous cell carcinoma
Tuberculosis
Syphilitic gummata

HYPERPIGMENTATION

Freckles
Chloasma
Pregnancy
Neurofibromatosis

Cushing's disease
Haemochromatosis

Addison's disease

DEPIGMENTATION

Vitiligo   Albinism

PLAQUES

Psoriasis   Lichen planus
Seborrhoeic dermatitis   Paget's disease of the nipple
Atopic dermatitis   Lupus erythematosus

HYPERKERATOSIS

Corns   Ichthyosis

VEGETATIVE

Warts   Condylomata
Squamous cell carcinoma

ATROPHY

Senile skin   Lupus erythematosus
Scleroderma

When the *nature* of the lesion has been established, its *characteristics* should be defined according to size, shape, surface and colour.

The next step is to discover the *distribution* of the rash. In some diseases, the diagnosis can be made from the distribution, and in others, it is of much assistance. The inference should not be drawn, however, that because a disease does not present itself in its common pattern of distribution, that it can be excluded. For example, psoriasis is commonly found on the extensors, but occasionally it will present itself as a solitary lesion in the external ear; a basal cell carcinoma is commonest on the face, but occasionally it occurs on the trunk. On the other hand, rosacea only attacks those areas of the face that flush.

The regional distribution of common conditions is as follows, and as will be seen, several diseases may overlap or occur simultaneously, but in different areas.

2. Distribution

SCALP

Seborrhoeic dermatitis   Alopecia

Psoriasis
Tinea

Sebaceous cysts
Pediculosis

FACE

Acne
Rosacea
Impetigo
Infantile eczema
Seborrhoeic dermatitis

Contact dermatitis
Sebaceous cysts
Neoplasms
Lupus erythematosus
Seborrhoeic warts

EYELIDS

Contact dermatitis
Warts

Xanthelasma
Neoplasms

LIPS

Herpes simplex
Cheilitis
Contact dermatitis

Neoplasms
Leukoplakia

MOUTH

Aphthous stomatitis
Leukoplakia
Lichen planus

Neoplasms
Pemphigus

EARS

Seborrhoeic dermatitis
Contact dermatitis
Otitis externa

Psoriasis
Lupus erythematosus
Neoplasm

CHEST

Acne
Seborrhoeic dermatitis
Pityriasis versicolor

Psoriasis
Pityriasis rosea
Seborrhoeic warts

AXILLAE

Contact dermatitis
Seborrhoeic dermatitis
Pediculosis

Boils
Tinea
Candidiasis

ABDOMEN
Pityriasis rosea
Psoriasis
Urticaria
Seborrhoeic warts

Drug eruptions
Candidiasis
Scabies

BACK
Acne
Seborrhoeic dermatitis
Psoriasis

Pityriasis rosea
Seborrhoeic warts

ANO-GENITAL AREA
Pruritus
Seborrhoeic dermatitis
Intertrigo
Tinea cruris (in males)
Scabies
Warts
Candidiasis

Contact dermatitis
Psoriasis
Pediculosis pubis
Syphilis
Herpes simplex
Lichen planus

HANDS
Contact dermatitis
Hyperidrosis
Dysidrosis

Warts
Scabies
Atopic dermatitis

ARMS
Psoriasis
Contact dermatitis

Lichen planus

LEGS
Contact dermatitis
Neurodermatitis
Varicose dermatitis
Psoriasis

Lichen planus
Purpura
Erythema nodosum
Insect bites

FEET
Tinea
Warts
Dysidrosis
Psoriasis

Contact dermatitis
Atopic dermatitis
Corns

Apart from these visible signs, there are in some conditions other aids to diagnosis.

1. *Patch tests* are described on page 55, in connection with contact dermatitis.

2. *Laboratory tests* to exclude fungus or bacterial infection. Special studies, such as an examination of the blood for L.E. cells, in lupus erythematosus, and platelet abnormalities in purpuric conditions. Other more routine tests, such as blood counts, sedimentation rates, and urine analyses may have to be carried out.

3. *Biopsy* is required in some chronic dermatoses, in all pigmented lesions which have been excised (see pigmented naevi) and in any conditions suspected of malignancy.

Biopsy

In most cases, it is best to select a fully developed lesion. In vesicular, bullous or pustular lesions, very early lesions are preferable, as otherwise secondary changes such as infection may make diagnosis extremely difficult.

Normal tissue should generally not be included unless a large specimen is being taken by the technician for processing. It is important to include subcutaneous fat, as diagnostic features may be found there.

Under aseptic conditions, and with local anaesthesia, the chosen piece is excised and the wound sutured. The specimen is placed on a piece of paper, smoothed out and allowed to dry for a minute or so, then, with the paper attached, put in a bottle containing 10 per cent formol saline, for transport to the laboratory.

Prior to biopsy or other surgical procedures, such as curettage of warts, it is advisable to obtain written permission for the operation from the patient or relatives.

Having taken the history, and identified the lesions, it is well to have in mind a tentative classification of disease. At first, many of the names of skin diseases sound strange, but familiarity with them soon dispels dismay.

A useful broad general classification is that of:

1. Inflammatory, scaly and infectious.
2. Granulomatous.
3. Neoplastic.

The first group includes those in chapters 6–14; the second group, lupus erythematosus, tuberculosis and sarcoidosis, and the third, the conditions described in chapter 20.

A sound diagnosis depends on acute observation of the lesions and an accurate history, culminating in their careful integration.

CHAPTER 3

Treatment

Dermatological treatment is no more complicated than that of any other specialty.

It should consist of treatment of the patient and the disease. It is extremely easy to forget the patient in the course of one's zeal to identify a lesion, either because of lack of time or because one considers the condition so trivial that it can safely be considered in isolation. Some patients are apparently less affected by skin diseases than others, whereas a disproportionate degree of concern may be a clue to some unmentioned problem with mind or body, and one must discover how much *the patient* is affected, in order to judge the amount of attention he, himself, should receive, as opposed to the disease. Some patients, for example, show a sense of profound revulsion as owners of a wart, or (in the case of women) of downy hair on the upper lip, whilst others have a more balanced attitude. Successful end-results can be obtained in treating only the lesions, but it is far more satisfying for both doctor (and patient) to treat both patient and disease.

GENERAL CONSIDERATIONS

In any discussion of the treatment of skin diseases, it should be stated that the most important ingredient, as in the treatment of diseases of other systems, is commonly *rest*. Patients find it extremely difficult to believe that rest will be very beneficial as, except for the irritation and the appearance of the rash, they are not much physically handicapped. If they are told, however, that the tissue of the skin differs little in its reaction to disease and rest, from affections of, for example, the lungs or stomach, the necessity for rest may be more easily understood. They should also be told that rest very definitely reduces the amount of itching, which is so vulnerable to environmental changes, and, when in an inflamed condition, to the petty stresses of daily life.

In generalized inflammatory conditions, the patient must be put to bed, and no compromise, such as lying on a couch, should be considered. The good effects of bed-rest are quickly visible. The only exception is that old people should be allowed to sit out of bed for longer periods daily. In their case the avoidance of the development of broncho-pneumonia and bed-sores easily outweighs the consideration that additional ambulation may prolong treatment.

Less aged patients should be allowed to go to the toilet when necessary, and sit up for a little while every day.

Anti-boredom devices are essential for otherwise active patients, and good sisters and nurses are adept in providing these.

Diet has little place in skin diseases, with the possible exception of slimming for the obese with either intertrigo or leg ulcers. Some patients with acne find that pastries and other confections provoke the appearance of lesions. Some with rosacea find that alcohol and hot or spicy liquids do the same. Sensitivity to food is a rare cause of skin disease, but when it is, the offending item must be proscribed.

Treatment of the disease can be divided into:

> (a) prophylactic measures;
> (b) curative measures.

(A) PROPHYLACTIC MEASURES

Prophylactic measures can be adopted in any particular disease by avoiding substances or conditions which are known to provoke an eruption.

Examples are the avoidance of sunlight when light-exposed areas are affected, as in lupus erythematosus; the restriction of shaving, when the beard area is infected; the avoidance of long periods of standing or sitting, when varicose dermatitis is present; or withdrawal from situations known to cause contact dermatitis.

(B) CURATIVE MEASURES

> (a) local, or external;
> (b) general, or internal.

External Treatment

A good general rule is to apply wet dressings or lotions to oozing lesions, and creams, ointments or pastes to dry lesions. If an ointment is applied to an oozing lesion, the exudate will force it from the area being treated, thus nullifying any potential benefits it might provide. Medicated baths are also sometimes useful.

The absorption rate of drugs is determined largely by their lipid/water partition coefficients; the main problem is the penetration of the epidermal keratin, which forms a barrier to the penetration of water-soluble substances; the dermis is freely permeable. As would be surmised, from their lipid solubility, steroids and sex hormones diffuse readily into the skin after topical application, and they are also metabolized there.

If the drug is water soluble, systemic administration is usually necessary. Anti-fungal and anti-bacterial agents are often more effective, therefore, when given by other routes.

Investigations are constantly directed towards developing inert organic solvents that might facilitate drug penetration through the skin, but up to now, they have met with limited success.

External treatment will be dealt with under the headings set out below.

(A) DRESSINGS

Those most commonly used are:

1. *Normal saline:* 5 g of salt to half a litre of water. This is the simplest to use.
2. *Potassium permanganate* solution in water: 1/8,000.
3. *Liquor aluminium acetate* (Burow's solution): 5 ml to half a litre of water.

Their *action* is antipruritic and cooling, and they soften crusts; to maintain these effects, they must be kept damp.

Their *indication* is that of acute inflammation, such as acute contact or atopic dermatitis, when vesicles, pustules, and oozing lesions exist.

The *method of application* is to soak layers of cotton or unstarched linen in the cool solution. The dressing is gently wrung out, applied damp to the lesions, and kept in place by a hand towel. The outer layers of cotton or linen are constantly removed, dampened, and reapplied to maintain a moist dressing.

(B) BATHS

The most useful are:

1. *Tar*, for psoriasis. About 100 ml of liquor picis carbonis are added to a bath, in which the patient should lie for at least ten minutes. Polytar emollient (Stiefel) is also effective.

2. *Potassium permanganate*, 1/8,000 solution in water, is useful for itchy, infected or eczematous conditions of the hands or feet, although this has a tendency to produce a rather dry skin.

3. *Emulsifying bath*, for infants with eczema. Add 10–20 g of emulsifying ointment B.P. to an infant-sized bath of about 45 litres.

4. *Oilatum oil* (*Stiefel*). This is effective, and easy to use.

(C) POLYTHENE COVERINGS

These may be particularly useful in psoriasis, chronic eczema, or localized neurodermatitis or lichen planus or pompholyx.

Polythene lay-flat tubing is a seamless plastic tube sold in various widths and gauges to accommodate the arms, legs, or trunk.

The cream or ointment to be used (usually a steroid in these cases) is applied fairly liberally, the polythene is then put on and made airtight around the ends with adhesive tape or elastic bands. The dressings are left untouched for 24 hours unless there is much discomfort from the heat and/or moisture which develop. Sometimes, it may only be possible for the patient to wear such a dressing at night. Steroid intoxication must be considered (see p. 30).

(D) POWDERS

These have protective and absorptive properties, and may also be antipruritic or astringent. Starch, talcum, and zinc oxide are common ingredients. They are useful for lesions in creases, such as the groins. They must be cautiously applied to weeping and raw surfaces.

An example of a basic powder is: zinc, starch and talc dusting-powder B.P.C. This contains one part of zinc oxide and starch to two of talc.

(E) LOTIONS

These are solutions or suspensions in water, or spirit.

1. *Calamine lotion*
This contains Calamine (zinc carbonate), zinc oxide, and glycerin in distilled water. It is apt to be too drying but is useful for insect bites, or urticaria.

2. *Oily calamine lotion*
This is used when the first type causes too much drying. It contains calamine with various oils in a solution of calcium hydroxide.

3. *Steroid lotions*
A great number of proprietary forms are now used. Half per cent strength is often as useful as 2 per cent. Preparations may also incorporate an antibiotic, and are used in this manner when an infective element exists. Steroids in any form have become the most useful weapons in dealing with itchy dermatoses. Their use is greatly enhanced if their potential dangers are continually kept in mind, and their employment carefully chosen.

These lotions are best used when small areas are involved; when they are large, steroid sprays may be tried. They are most useful in pruritus ani and vulvae, contact, atopic and neuro-dermatitis.

The following are a few examples of proprietary brands of steroid lotions: with hydrocortisone (Efcortelan), with betamethasone (Betnovate), with fluocinolone (Synalar) and with triamcinolone (Adcortyl).

4. *Zinc sulphide lotion B.N.F.*
This contains sulphurated potash and zinc sulphate in camphor water, and is one of the most useful local remedies for acne.

5. *Salicylic Acid Lotion B.P.C.*
This contains:

Salicylic acid	2 g
Castor oil	1 ml
Industrial methylated spirit to	100 ml

Labelling: Caution. This preparation is inflammable. Keep away from a naked flame. It is useful for seborrhoea.

(F) OINTMENTS AND PASTES

Ointments consist of animal, mineral, or vegetable oils as bases, and in these various substances are incorporated. Ointments may thus be made anti-pruritic, antiseptic, astringent, or given whatever quality is required.

Pastes are mixtures of powders and ointments. They are thicker, more protective, and more adherent than ointments, and therefore more difficult to apply and remove. The use of ointments and pastes is restricted, creams being preferred whenever possible.

The following are used as bases for ointments:

(a) White paraffin
(b) Lanolin
(c) Carbowax
(d) Emulsifying ointment

Examples of medicated ointments and pastes are as follows:

1. Whitfield's ointment

Salicylic acid	1 g	3%
Benzoic acid	2 g	6%
Carbowax to	30 g	91%

This is used chiefly for fungal infections of the feet. It has been superseded by less messy remedies (e.g. Tinaderm cream) to a large extent, and also by griseofulvin tablets (see Chapter 10).

2. Calamine ointment

Calamine	5 g	16·7%
White soft paraffin	25 g	83·3%

This is used for chronic dry itchy dermatoses.

3. Some proprietary antibiotic ointments:

tetracyline (Achromycin), chlortetracycline (Aureomycin), oxytetracycline (Terramycin), sodium fusidate (Fucidin).

They are very useful in infected conditions such as impetigo, or folliculitis; the organism should be identified and its drug sensitivity solved before prescribing the appropriate ointment.

It should be noted that penicillin ointment or cream must never be used on the skin, because of the great risk of sensitization, resulting in a dermatitis which is extremely difficult to cure. The same applies to sulphonamide and antihistamine ointments and creams. Neomycin and the chemically related Framycetin may also sensitize the skin, especially in eczematous subjects, and particularly when used in an ointment base; if its use is unavoidable, it should be in the form of a cream or powder.

There are many proprietary brands of steroid ointments, as there are creams (see below). They contain 0·05–2·5 per cent of the active agent.

(G) CREAMS

These are soft ointments, usually composed of bases containing a high proportion of water, liquid paraffin, or arachis oil.

Examples are:

1. Calamine Cream B.P.C. Used for inflammatory conditions.
2. Zinc Cream B.P.C. Also for inflammatory conditions, or as a vehicle for tar.
3. Crem. Zinc. et Ol. Ricin. B.P. Zinc and castor oil. Used mainly for infants.
4. Hydrocortisone Cream B.P.C. 1 per cent in a water soluble base. There are many proprietary brands of steroid creams; e.g. with fluocinolone (Synalar), with betamethasone (Betnovate), with clobetasol propionate (Dermovate), and with fluocinonide (Metosyn). These are stronger than hydrocortisone and are the most effective steroid creams. Many steroid creams are also made containing antibiotics, e.g. Betnovate with aureomycin. Some incorporate tar, e.g. Tarcortin, Clioquinol, Dioderm C, and some contain both, e.g. Cor-tar-quin.

One must be constantly aware of the toxic effects of such powerful agents as clobetasol propionate and betamethasone valerate, which manifest themselves, apart from signs of general steroid intoxication, as atrophy and/or telangiectasia of the treated areas.

They may be very effective in the following conditions:

Atopic dermatitis: for relatively small areas.

Contact dermatitis: for small areas, but less useful than in atopic dermatitis.

Localized neurodermatitis.
Pruritus ani and vulvae.
Nummular eczema.
Psoriasis.

(H) ANTIPRURITICS
The following are the best:
Steroids   Tar
Calamine

(I) ANTISEPTICS
The following are the best:
Potassium permanganate
Cetrimide (Cetavlon)
Eusol (contains calcium hypochlorite and boric acid)
Iodochlorhydroxyquinoline (Vioform). Constant use can occasionally
cause hypothyroidism.

(J) PAINTS
These are occasionally used on areas where creases exist, such as the
anogenital areas or between the toes.

1. Magenta Paint B.P.C.
This contains magenta, phenol, boric acid and resorcinol amongst
other substances.
    It is useful as an antipruritic, and also for its drying effects on
moist lesions in the anogenital area, and between the toes.
    It stains clothing, and should be stored in the dark.

2. Coal Tar Paint B.P.C.
    Crude coal tar   10 g
    Acetone
    Benzene of, equal volumes to 100 ml
It is used predominantly in lichenified dermatitis and psoriasis. It is
inflammable.

3. Podophyllin Compound Paint B.P.C.
2–5 per cent podophyllin in Tinct. Benz. Co. is useful for anogenital
warts, and plantar warts.
    This paint is very irritating to the eyes.

The table below shows the quantities of preparations it is advisable to prescribe.

	Creams and Ointments (g)	Lotions (ml)
Face	25	100
Hands	50	250
Scalp	50	250
Arms and legs	100	250
Body	200	500
Groins and genitalia	25	100
Dusting Powders	50 or 100 g	
Paints	10 or 20 ml	

Internal Treatment

There are only a few drugs but these benefit a disproportionate number of dermatoses.

The drugs are:

    (a) Steroids
    (b) Antibiotics
    (c) Antihistamines
    (d) Anti-malarials
    (e) Endocrines
    (f) Immunosuppressants
    (g) Vitamins
    (h) Sedatives

(A) STEROIDS

The discovery of cortisone has revolutionized the treatment of many dermatoses, as it has done in the management of conditions previously unmanageable in other branches of medicine. As should be known, they are double-edged weapons, capable of doing as much harm as good. In certain dermatoses, such as pemphigus, and systemic lupus erythematosus, their life-saving, or life-prolonging qualities, far outweigh any consideration of the harm they can do. In many non-fatal conditions, however, in which they produce remarkable improvements, there may be a tendency to prescribe them without duly weighing the pros and cons.

In benign conditions, the following points should be considered: (1) are steroids the most effective treatment? (2) for how long must they be given?

The recognized contra-indications to the giving of steroids are:

1. Chronic nephritis
2. Cardiac failure
3. Peptic ulcer
4. Coronary thrombosis of recent origin
5. Diabetes mellitus
6. Senile osteoporosis

The following conditions are those in which steroids have been found to be useful, and may be given after due consideration:

1. Atopic dermatitis
2. Contact dermatitis
3. Erythema nodosum
4. Exfoliative dermatitis
5. Lichen planus
6. Lupus erythematosus: (a) systemic, (b) localized
7. Pemphigus
8. Urticaria; when acute, a short course may be justified

Steroids in ointments and lotions have already been dealt with (*vide supra*).

(B) ANTIBIOTICS

(i) (*Broad-spectrum*) such as tetracycline (Achromycin) or oxytetracycline (Terramycin) or erythromycin. They are given in tablet or capsule form. They may be used in:

Acne
Boils
Carbuncles
Inflammatory dermatoses complicated by infection.

Although acne lesions are sterile, the oxytetracycline group of antibiotics often produce the most satisfying results, for reasons unknown; and relatively small doses can be given for long periods (see p. 211). This also applies to rosacea. Apart from symptoms of nausea and/or diarrhoea whilst taking these antibiotics, ano-

genital pruritus, although uncommon, is a complication of which to
be wary.

(ii) (*Narrow-spectrum*) such as griseofulvin.

GRISOVIN

is an antibiotic obtained by the fermentation of several species of
penicillin.

It is extremely effective in most types of superficial fungus disease;
in fact, against all known species of Microsporum, Trichophyton
and Epidermophyton. It is not effective against Candida albicans.
The antibiotic is fungistatic, and not fungicidal.

Its greatest value is in ringworm of the scalp and chronic infections
of the skin and nails.

This drug is given as a tablet of 125 mg or 500 mg. The tablets
are best taken altogether and not in divided lots, after the main
meal of the day. For dosages, see Chapter 10. Treatment in chronic
nail infections may have to last a year or more. Severe reactions are
rare, but reversible side-effects such as diarrhoea, headache, leucopenia or albuminuria may occur. Its safety in pregnancy has not
been established, and is contraindicated in patients with porphyria,
and severe liver disease.

(C) ANTIHISTAMINES

These may be given by mouth in tablets of varying strengths, 3 times
daily, according to the proprietary tablet. Examples are: triprolidine hydrochloride (Actidil) 2·5 mg, and chlorpheniramine maleate
(Piriton) 4 mg. The most important side effect is drowsiness.

They are used predominantly in urticaria.

They must not be given topically, as the sensitization rate is high.

Contraindications are (1) epilepsy, (2) early pregnancy, (3) those
already receiving mainly synergistic drugs.

(D) ANTI-MALARIALS

Nivaquine (Chloroquine Sulphate). This is sometimes effective in
chronic lupus erythematosus. 200 mg tablets twice daily is the usual
initial dose, which is later reduced.

Toxic symptoms are not uncommon, and vary from pruritus and
diarrhoea to serious ocular complications such as amblyopia (see

treatment of chronic lupus erythematosus). Regular ophthalmic examination is essential in those taking this drug for a long time.

(E) ENDOCRINES

The contraceptive pill is often beneficial in acne. Side-effects are not uncommon, especially that of increased pigmentation of the forehead, lower parts of the cheeks and areas above the upper lip. Other side-effects are, acne, genital candidiasis, telangiectases, photosensitivity, and small patches of eczema on various sites. Acne may become worse at the onset of treatment, but this should not inhibit the continuation of treatment, providing there are no side-effects.

(F) IMMUNOSUPPRESSANTS

Those drugs which are folic acid antagonists are now used for several skin diseases, in the form of methotrexate. They block DNA synthesis in the nucleus, preventing cell division. They have therefore come into use in psoriasis, in which epidermal cells reproduce rapidly, and in pemphigus vulgaris and pemphigoid, which at the present time are thought to be auto-immune diseases.

Toxicity from the drug is manifested in normal tissues that are characterized by high rates of mitotic activity, i.e. tissues that require large quantities of nucleoproteins, namely oral and gastric mucosa, hair matrix, and normal bone marrow. Side-effects consist of stomatitis, temporary alopecia, leuco- and thrombocytopenia, these last two symptoms depending on the size of the dosage; anorexia, nausea, malaise, headaches and diarrhoea, also occur. Smallpox vaccination may be hazardous during treatment, while long-term dangers involve the liver and central nervous system.

(G) VITAMINS

Vitamin A is sometimes useful in ichthyosis. Otherwise vitamins are given for general rather than specific effects.

(H) SEDATIVES

These may be essential to allay itching, particularly at night, when the work of a day's treatment may be undone, although daytime sedation is also sometimes required.

For daytime, the following may be given: Valium (diazepam) 5–10 mg three times a day, or Librium (chlordiazepoxide) 5–10 mg three times a day or Stelazine 1 mg (trifluoperazine).

For night time, give Tuinal 200 mg, Nembutal 200 mg or Mogadon (nitrazepam) 5 mg.

Physical Agents

Apart from the measures described above physical agents (see, for example, Fig. 2) are also used in the therapy of skin diseases.

They are:
diathermy   X-rays
cautery   Grenz rays
carbon dioxide   dermabrasion
ultra-violet rays

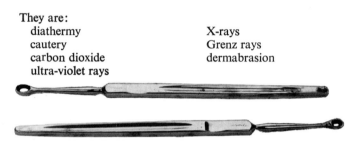

FIG. 2. Curettes, for the removal of warts.

CAUTERY AND DIATHERMY

With both these methods an electrified needle destroys the lesion with which it is in contact (Fig. 3).

Both methods are used for destroying common warts, seborrhoeic warts, senile keratoses, certain naevi, and basal cell carcinomata.

CRYOTHERAPY

Carbon dioxide is the most commonly used freezing agent. It is obtained easily by means of a 'Sparklet' machine, in which single cylinders emit the gas through a small hole into a collecting tube. This appears as solid snow.

It may be used as (a) a solid stick, its effect depending on the pressure and duration of the application or (b) in the form of a slush, which is obtained when the stick is mixed with acetone.

(a) Its use in the form of a stick is for the treatment of plantar warts, seborrhoeic warts and senile keratoses.

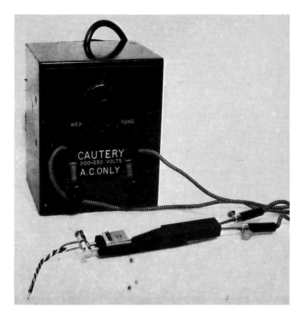

FIG. 3. Cautery machine, handle and point.

(b) In the form of slush when combined with a few drops of acetone, it is employed on patches of chronic lupus erythematosus, and chronic exuberant acne lesions.

Liquid nitrogen is another form of cryotherapy. A cotton wool swab is saturated with the liquid and applied to the lesion for 5–15 seconds, depending on its size and depth. It is useful for treating common and plantar warts, although the latter need a somewhat longer application.

ULTRA-VIOLET RAYS

Indications are: acne and psoriasis.

Contra-indications are: lupus erythematosus, photo-sensitive eruptions, and a history of pulmonary tuberculosis.

X-RAYS

X-rays are of various energies and types. They may be regulated so that they do not penetrate the skin; a practice not followed in the days of their use for scalp ringworm, a failure of which the later development of brain tumours has been evidence.

The usefulness of X-rays is declining, and cases must be carefully selected.

Indications are:

    acne, in some carefully selected cases
    basal cell carcinoma
    circumscribed neurodermatitis
    otitis externa
    seborrhoeic dermatitis, when localized to intertriginous areas

GRENZ RAYS

These have less penetrating potential than X-rays, and therefore potentially less dangerous.

They are used for:
    lichen planus
    psoriasis
    circumscribed neurodermatitis

DERMABRASION

Its use has diminished greatly in the U.K. in recent years. The skin is abraded with a device similar to a dentist's drill, the drill being replaced by a wire-brush mandrel. When in vogue, it was used for acne scarring, and superficial forms of haemangiomata.

It will be observed from the foregoing pages of this chapter, that whilst most skin diseases are curable or controllable, the exact mode of action of the drug used is commonly obscure. Why sulphur is topically useful in acne and seborrhoea, and steroids in pemphigus, for example, is not understood. The use of most drugs in dermatology is empiric, that is, treatment is based on the results of experience, rather than scientific knowledge. If the contra-indications and the complications of drug therapy are known, however, the experienced physician should have little difficulty in the management of skin diseases.

CHAPTER 4

Eczema and Dermatitis

Atopic Eczema: Discoid Eczema: Pompholyx
Contact Dermatitis

More than half of all skin diseases fall under this heading. Both terms denote an acute, subacute, or chronic inflammatory condition, characterized by:

1. Erythema and oedema;
2. Discrete or grouped vesicles, progressing to weeping and crusted lesions, with or without papules and scaling;
3. Itching or burning, causing scratching or rubbing, which later leads to lichenification (thickening) of the skin.

Both terms, eczema and dermatitis, are used synonymously.

The cause of eczema or dermatitis is, on the one hand, external or traumatic, and, on the other hand, internal or constitutional. When external causes are responsible the condition is called contact dermatitis. When internal causes are responsible, four principal varieties of eczema or dermatitis may be produced:

1. Atopic eczema
2. Nummular eczema
3. Pompholyx
4. Seborrhoeic dermatitis (p. 71)

Atopic Eczema

Atopic Dermatitis; Allergic Eczema; Besnier's Prurigo;
Disseminated Neurodermatitis

Atopy is a term used to describe the following phenomena:

1. A marked familial tendency to allergic diseases such as asthma, hay-fever, urticaria, and rhinitis.

2. A high degree of hypersensitivity to protein substances.

3. Nervous system disturbances reflected by unusual reactions to heat, cold, and emotional tensions.

Atopic eczema is frequently associated with these phenomena. The atopy is separate from the eczema, as can be shown by the fact that if it transpires that the patient is sensitive to a certain type of food, the giving of it, or its deprivation, will not affect the eczema one way or another.

About 10 per cent of the general population suffer from atopic disorders, but not all suffer from eczema. About 3 per cent of all infants suffer from atopic eczema. A family history is present in about 70 per cent of all cases.

PATHOLOGY

The acute phase is characterized by oedema in the epidermis. Varying degrees of acanthosis also occur. As the condition progresses and becomes more chronic, hyperkeratosis and parakeratosis follow. The dermis invariably shows a perivascular infiltrate. The changes are non-specific.

CLINICAL FEATURES

These vary with the age of the patient, and occur as three varieties.

1. *Infantile Eczema*

The time of onset is usually about the second month. The skin is red, with small vesicles on a puffy surface, and small cracks ooze serum (Fig. 4). The sites commonly attacked are the face, except for the skin around the mouth, nose, and eyes; the forearms, wrists, outer parts of the legs, and the flexures. Recovery usually occurs between the third and fourth year after periods of remissions and relapses, although a small percentage of cases clear up in the first 18 months.

A non-atopic variety of infantile eczema occasionally occurs, which responds to treatment, and does not last more than a few weeks. If it does do so, it shows itself to be of the atopic type, although a small percentage of cases clears up in the first 18 months.

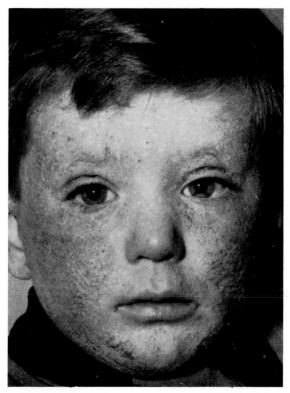

FIG. 4. Infantile eczema. Crusting and scaling, with the characteristic relative freedom of the circumoral area. The worried expression is also typical.

2. *Childhood Type*

This may follow directly from the infantile variety, form a recurrence, or appear for the first time. Papular and lichenoid lesions are commonest, and the flexor surfaces are those most often affected. Lesions usually disappear by the age of 10 or 12.

3. *Adult Type*

This may or may not be preceded by a history of infantile eczema. and/or the childhood type. The lesions are papular and lichenified and excoriations are common. Crusting and exudation follow scratching.

The sites commonly attacked are the flexures, and then the front and sides of the neck, eyelids, forehead, face, chest, wrists, and the backs of the feet and the hands. In mild cases, only one or two areas may be affected. The course is intermittent and there may be relatively long periods of freedom from lesions, although chronicity is the rule.

Other Findings

Ichthyosis (page 253) affects about 10 per cent of patients with atopic eczema. It does not improve when the eczema does.

Itching is severe, and a change in room temperature, a change in mood, or friction from wool is enough to irritate the skin.

Sweat retention is often marked. *Chronic secondary bacterial infection* is common.

A tense or aggressive *mental attitude* is often noted.

A certain proportion of patients with atopic eczema develop *juvenile ocular cataracts*.

No young patient with this disease must be vaccinated because of the danger of *eczema vaccinatum* (vaccinia superimposed on eczema), which in its severest form causes death. Nor should they have contact with others who have active vaccinia lesions. Adults must be carefully assessed before being vaccinated.

DIAGNOSIS

This is made by the character and distribution of the lesions, the itching, and the family and allergic history.

The disease must be distinguished from *contact dermatitis* in which itching is inconstant and the lesions are relatively localized, any area being affected. In *seborrhoeic dermatitis* the lesions are not particularly itchy and are not on flexor surfaces. *Localized neurodermatitis* is characterized by well-circumscribed, occasional and itchy lesions on any area.

TREATMENT

This condition calls for more skill and patience on the part of the physician than any other skin disease.

Sympathy and understanding are an enormous help to the patient (and parents), and even an intimation of pessimism or despair may have disastrous consequences. It is important that the patient or parents should know about the course and consequences of the disease.

There is no specific therapy but a great deal can be done to help these difficult cases.

Prophylactic measures

Sudden changes of temperature must be avoided, such as undressing in a cold atmosphere or entering too hot a bath. In summer, light clothing should be worn at night and a well-ventilated room is essential. Irritating clothing, such as woollens, or sharp straps, or buckles attached to clothing, must not be worn, and soaps, detergents, and other household cleansers must be avoided so far as possible.

Pillows and mattresses should be made of foam rubber, and regular hours of sleep (and meals) are advisable.

Curative measures

For the *acute* or moist forms of the disease (or any dermatitis) Burow's solution (aluminium acetate), calamine lotion, or a steroid lotion or spray are useful provided that care is taken to prevent over-drying of the skin which produces fissures; should they occur, they will be resolved by the use of creams. Emulsifying baths are also very useful in this acute phase (see p. 27).

For the *chronic* or dry forms of the disease, applications of steroid creams can help, and when extra penetrative effect is required, they may be applied under a polythene covering; steroid intoxication can occur with this technique (p. 30). Sometimes these preparations fail to relieve or improve the condition, and other ointments, such as 2 per cent liquor picis carbonis in zinc ointment can be tried.

N.B. Antihistamine preparations must not be prescribed (see p. 34).

Systemic therapy in the form of steroids may be given only in severe cases and after much thought. Although the improvement is dramatic the chief drawback is that when the drug is withdrawn, inflammation may recur in a form more furious than before, which could nullify the progress of the day. It should, therefore, only be used for either extremely or extensively involved, and disabled patients. It should not be given to children.

Sedation at night should be given to reduce scratching.

Psychotherapy as a supportive measure in the treatment of atopic dermatitis is important, although it should not be one of the main methods of treatment. When confidential rapport between doctor and patient has been established, conditions of stress at home or at work should be discussed, and an optimistic prognosis put forward. Moreover, in the case of a sick child, the parents should be advised to refrain from acts of unconscious disgust towards the disease, in the form of acute anxiety to get rid of their child's disfigurement, or discussing the handicap he or she has to endure, especially in the child's hearing. Treatment by a psychiatrist is rarely if ever indicated, and such aid is generally not of much help.

Environmental change to hospital, or the home of a relative or friend, invariably produces a turn for the better, and this may reflect vague but real problems encountered in the home situation.

The overall aim in treatment, in fact, is to soothe by a combination of suitable applications, the avoidance of physical and/or psychological stress, and the indoctrination of hope and confidence in the outcome, as opposed to the destructive effects of melancholy.

Discoid Eczema (Nummular Eczema)

This chronic inflammatory condition is characterized by coin-shaped or nummular lesions, which may be dry or wet. It occurs at any age, but particularly in tense, middle-aged individuals. It may also be present as a manifestation of atopic eczema in infants and children under 10.

CAUSE

This is unknown. It can be seen at any age, particularly in tense middle-aged individuals. It may also present as a manifestation of atopic dermatitis in infants and children under the age of 10.

PATHOLOGY

The picture is one of acute or chronic dermatitis.

CLINICAL SIGNS

Itching is common, and sometimes intense. The onset is insidious, and at first there are only one or two lesions, but they multiply. The lesions are papular, and consist of very small vesicles, which soon burst, leaving crusts. The lesions usually coalesce to form plaques. Any site may be affected, but more commonly on the back of the hands and forearms, the calves and the front of the thighs.

COURSE

This is difficult to predict, some cases clearing within a month or two, others following an indolent course of remissions and relapses for a year or more.

DIAGNOSIS

This disorder must be distinguished from *ringworm* whose lesions have a red margin with scaling, while the centre shows healing. In *psoriasis* there are no vesicles, and itching is absent.

TREATMENT

The same topical and internal measures are used as for atopic dermatitis. These may be supplemented by diazepam (Valium) tabs. 5 mg t.d.s. or other transquillizers when indicated.

Natural sunlight is useful, while cold weather and too many baths must be avoided.

Pompholyx

Dysidrosis

This is an acute or subacute disorder of the hands (cheiropompholyx) and/or the feet (pedopompholyx), characterized by deep-seated itchy vesicles. Pompholyx can be considered to be an unusual type of eczema or dermatitis.

Pompholyx may be caused by excessive sweating of the affected areas, with emotional upsets, with tinea of the feet, and occasionally with contact dermatitis.

PATHOLOGY

The vesicles are intra-epidermal, and often independent of the sweat-duct. There are few or no inflammatory changes to be seen.

CLINICAL SIGNS

Itching and burning sensations are usual, and occur most severely as a new lesion is being formed. The onset may be gradual or sudden. Lesions are vesicular, similar to boiled sago grains. The surface is at first smooth, but later, when the vesicle has ruptured, a brownish scale develops. The lesion has white overtones owing to its contents, and the surrounding skin usually shows little change. Sometimes this renders them difficult to see.

Sites: the sides of the fingers, the palms, and the soles are attacked. In severe cases all these areas may be involved, in mild ones perhaps only a few lesions will be found on the fingers. The distribution is invariably bilateral. The nails in chronic cases are deformed.

DIAGNOSIS

The itching and character of the lesions are unmistakable, but the most important task in these cases is to discover the cause. *Tinea*, *contact dermatitis*, and *pustular psoriasis* should be considered in the diagnosis.

TREATMENT

If the cause is known and treated, the lesions clear up. But all too often it remains hidden, and symptomatic and empirical treatments have to be used.

External

Potassium permanganate 1/8,000 warm baths for the hands and/or feet b.d. for 10 minutes each, followed by the application of zinc or steroid cream which can be covered with polythene to increase its effect. X-rays may help in chronic cases.

Internal

Oral steroids may have to be used in very chronic cases.

PROGNOSIS

Recurrences are not uncommon. The interval between them varies between months and years.

Contact Dermatitis

Dermatitis venenata, occupational or industrial dermatitis

This condition is characterized by redness, oedema, vesicles, and sometimes bullae, and a variable amount of itching. It is caused by chemical or vegetable substances coming into contact with the skin.

About 10 per cent of dermatological patients attending hospital suffer from this disease, although of course this figure is variable and may well be higher in industrial areas and lower in rural ones.

CAUSE

Apart from the actual provoking cause, other factors are present. These are individual susceptibility, or conditions such as minor trauma, excessive sweating, atopic dermatitis or ichthyosis. Any of these in the mildest form can also be causative agents.

The actual cause may be either a *primary irritant*, or a *sensitizer*. In these cases one may speak of primary irritant dermatitis and allergic contact dermatitis, respectively. A *primary irritant* is a substance, such as lime or nitric acid, which will produce inflammation on first contact with the skin, if permitted to act in sufficient intensity or quantity for a sufficient time. The rash produced by primary irritants is self-limited, and disappears reasonably rapidly. Prevention of a recurrence is easy, once the irritant is recognized, by means of special clothing, washing after exposure, and barrier creams.

Sensitizers, such as flour, or dyes, are a much larger problem. The number of exposures to the substance necessary to cause a rash varies from a few to many. One baker, for example, will suddenly become sensitized to flour after handling it for years; another, following only a few exposures. This time factor varies incomprehensibly. Prevention is in most cases impossible, except by complete avoidance of contact with the offending substance.

Identification of the cause requires investigation of the patient's occupation, hobbies, household duties, wearing apparel, cosmetic articles, and holidays. The questions, though apparently exhaustive, may be fruitless. A daily diary may have to be kept by the patient, and in some cases, the work-bench or home surroundings visited by the physician.

Difficulties to be encountered may be gauged by the case of a woman who developed primula sensitivity in a friend's house, even though the plant was concealed behind a screen, or that of a clerk who worked for a market gardener and developed tomato sensitivity when he occasionally took a short cut through the greenhouse.

Just as important as a thorough investigation into the habits of the patient's life is (1) a knowledge of the special characteristics of substances causing contact dermatitis, and (2) acquaintance with the distribution of lesions caused by those substances.

1. SPECIAL CHARACTERISTICS OF SUBSTANCES CAUSING CONTACT DERMATITIS

The substances may be divided into the following groups:

(a) clothing,   (d) occupational,
(b) cosmetics,   (e) plants,
(c) household,   (f) medicines.

It will not be possible to mention here all substances, but it will be possible to give a guide to their miscellany.

(a) *Clothing*

The most common substances causing dermatitis in this category are organic dyes, rubber in elastic, and nickel in buttons, zips and hooks.

Dermatitis on the backs of the feet or toes may be caused by shoes, and be due to such constituents as resins, tar, plastic, leather or rubber.

Nylon stockings may cause a rash on the inner surface of the upper part of the thighs, backs of the knees, and on the feet and toes (Fig. 5). Nylon hair-nets may cause a rash on the back of the neck. In each case, the cause is generally a dye.

Nickel is one of the commonest causes of contact dermatitis, and is part of chromium-plated suspenders, zips, watch straps and buckles. Nickel is a very strong sensitizer and recovery often takes several years, interspersed with remissions and relapses. Although the areas in contact with nickel produce a dermatitis, it has an eccentric habit of secondarily attacking areas, such as the eyelids, and flexor surfaces of the elbows, which have never been in contact with it. The patient may therefore focus an unknowing doctor's attention on these areas, without informing him of a small patch, for example, under a suspender clip.

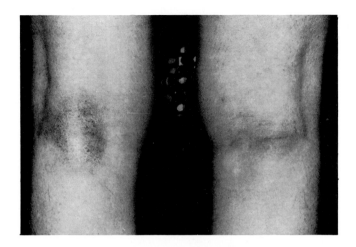

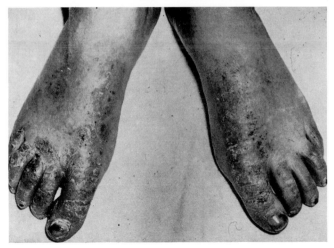

FIG. 5. Nylon dermatitis. Characteristic sites. The soles were also affected (Dr Harold Wilson).

Napkin dermatitis is one of the commonest skin diseases of infants. It is an erythematous and papulovesicular dermatitis, which occurs on the genitals, buttocks, thighs and lower abdomen, and in severe cases may spread to involve the chest and face, and legs and heels (Fig. 6).

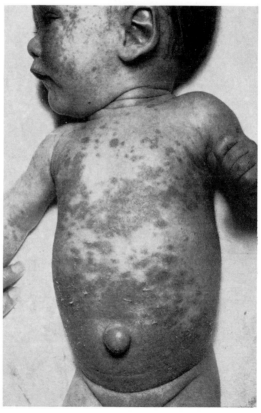

Fig. 6. General spread in a case of napkin dermatitis. There was no evidence of candidiasis.

It is usually due to prolonged wearing of wet napkins, and less often to the formation of ammonia in the wet napkin, as the result of the growth of a saprophytic bacillus splitting the urinary urea into ammonia; sometimes the cause may be candidiasis.

Disposable napkins should be used, the skin cleansed only with olive oil, and steroid creams or zinc and castor oil applied. The baby should be kept lying on its abdomen as much as possible.

(b) *Cosmetics*

Chemicals in cosmetics may cause primary irritant or sensitizing reactions, the latter being more common; irritating substances are usually removed by the manufacturers.

The commonest *sensitizers* are paraphenylenediamine, which is a hair dye, nail lacquers, perfumes, eye make-up preparations, preservatives (parabens) and lanolin.

Dermatitis due to cosmetics commonly affects the eyelids, neck and ears, and the area chiefly involved may not be that to which the cosmetic was applied; for example, mild hair-dye dermatitis may initially affect the eyelids; while in the case of nail polish the eyelids, neck and face may show a reaction, sparing the nail area.

Cosmetics most often associated with *irritant* reactions are antiperspirants, depilatories, and permanent wave preparations.

(c) *Household*

Detergents are a very common cause of dermatitis. They contain soap and synthetic detergents. When their cleaning action is considered it is not surprising to find that they can directly penetrate the horny layer, and defat the skin. The rash is usually most persistent, and may continue for a long time in spite of treatment. Very few patients can avoid doing household washing, the slightest amount of which is liable to cause the condition to bloom again. For many there is no economic alternative.

In comparison, other household substances play a small part, but such things as polishes and the wearing of rubber gloves can give rise to problems.

About half the cases of contact dermatitis are located on the hands. Of those which are occupational about 90 per cent are on the hands.

(d) *Occupational*

The number of causes under this heading is legion. The commonest

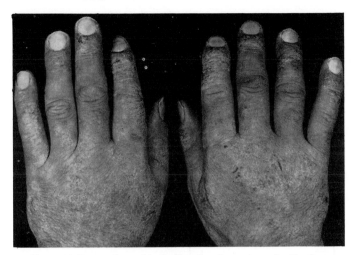

FIG. 7. (a) Cement dermatitis. Scaling, fissuring and crusting (Institute of Dermatology, University of London).

amongst them are petroleum products, oils, solvents, paint constituents and cement (Fig. 7a & b).

Less commonly, substances such as synthetic rubber, and natural rubber to which chemicals have been added, and natural or synthetic resins which are used in varnish and adhesives, may be the cause.

(e) *Plants*
The commonest plants responsible for dermatitis are primula, chrysanthemums, celery (Fig. 8), tulips and clematis. Daffodils and narcissi are the cause of many cases in the Scilly Isles, amongst pickers and packers.

(f) *Medicines*
The following drugs when applied to the skin are often the cause of dermatitis: penicillin, streptomycin, antihistamines, the procaine series of local anaesthetics, neomycin, framycetin and dequalinium chloride.

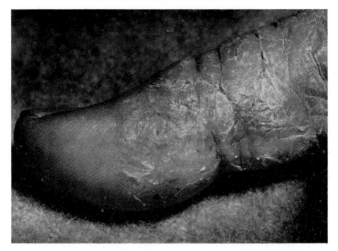

FIG. 7. (b) Cement dermatitis. Marked fissuring and scaling.

In some cases, however, contact with them is unavoidable. For example, nurses and doctors who are obliged to give injections are liable to have small quantities constantly falling on the skin. As the disease establishes itself, it may be impossible for the person to enter a room, a ward, or a theatre where particles of these drugs are in the atmosphere without developing an extremely itchy skin.

2. DISTRIBUTION OF LESIONS CAUSED BY OFFENDING SUBSTANCES

The head, neck, and face may be affected by cosmetics, and secondarily in the case of nickel dermatitis. Plants such as primula commonly produce lesions on the face.

The *hands* are the most commonly involved, so that the number of substances capable of causing dermatitis is enormous. Soap, detergents, petrol, oil and cement are some of the common causes.

The *arms* are most often affected by dusts and plants.

The *axillae* may be affected by cosmetics and clothing.

The *trunk* is usually involved by sensitization to such articles as metal clips, or elastic in underwear.

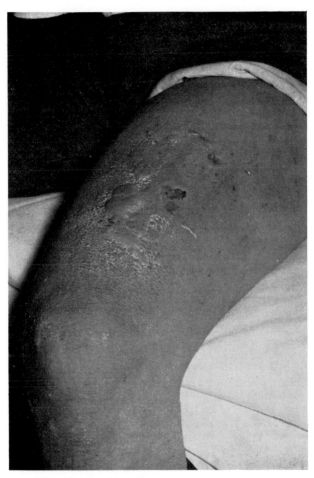

FIG. 8. Contact dermatitis. Bullae and vesicles following contact with celery leaves and exposure to sunlight. Also called phyto-photo-dermatitis. It may be caused by other plants, such as parsnips, or various weeds. Patient is a boy wearing short trousers.

The *feet* may present dermatitis caused by a constituent of shoes or socks. The dorsal surfaces of the feet, and not the soles, are affected.

These lists are not comprehensive, but should serve as a guide to one of the approaches in the diagnosis of the disease.

Patch Tests

When used correctly patch tests are invaluable in identifying sensitisers causing allergic contact dermatitis. A patch test is based on the assumption that if a substance causes dermatitis it should produce an inflammatory reaction when applied to an unaffected area of skin.

The method of performing the test is to apply some of the substance to the skin, and cover it with cellophane fixed in position with micropore or Scotch tape (Fig. 9). Several firms produce special adhesive tapes for testing, e.g., Dalmas, Neodermotest. Dilutions of the substance are made for the test. Reference for the specific dilutions must be made to a specialized work on the subject.

The test should be carried out during a quiescent phase of the dermatitis, otherwise a severe reaction may ensue. The patches should be placed in the middle of the back, as pigmentation may result and sometimes remain for months.

The patches are left in place for 48 hours, unless itching occurs before this time. Positive reactions of an allergic nature include inflammation and usually result in papules or vesicles. If negative after 48 hours they should be re-examined two days later. Some substances give positive patch tests only if the horny layer has been stripped from the area. This applies notably in Neomycin and antihistamine sensitivity.

A negative patch test reaction nearly always indicates an absence of allergic eczematous hypersensitivity to that particular substance. Whilst positive patch tests prove that the person is sensitive to the substance used for testing, the positive result must be judged in the light of all aspects of the case.

TREATMENT

Prophylactic

In industry, workers should be screened before being given jobs where dermatitis is a well-known risk. This is of course very difficult,

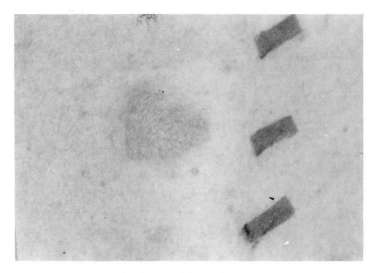

FIG. 9. Patch test showing a positive result, accompanied by a mild surrounding reaction to Scotch tape.

especially in small factories where medical facilities are slight or non-existent. Even in large building firms, for example, this is not done on account of the endless supply of labourers, so that cement dermatitis is not uncommon.

Working conditions must be good; protective clothing, such as gloves, and the existence of dust-extractors and efficient ventilators are examples of what may be done to reduce the chances of dermatitis.

In non-industrial cases, the patient must obviously avoid all contact with the offending substance. Again, it is more easily said than done, as in the case of housewife's dermatitis from soap and detergents.

Curative
The patient must be removed from the source of the dermatitis,

otherwise no treatment will cure it, and as a rule avoidance of the causative agent must be everlasting.

External measures for treating acute cases should consist only of absolutely bland applications, such as saline, Burow's solution, or potassium permanganate 1/8000 solution. Compresses, with old sheets or hand towels, for 5–10 minutes three times a day, followed by calamine lotion, are helpful.

Steroid preparations are not very efficacious in the most acute phase.

When the condition becomes less acute, it should be treated as for atopic dermatitis (p. 43).

Internal measures are sometimes necessary in the acute stages, and only in severe cases steroids should be considered. Their use often produces a dramatic result, but it must be remembered that they will not cure the disease if there is still contact with the offending substance.

Desensitization measures in contact dermatitis have always proved to be very difficult and disappointing.

PROGNOSIS

This depends on the primary cause and the possibility of avoiding exposure to it. Additional factors such as an atopic constitution and the patient's intelligence are also important. The prognosis is generally better in a case of sensitization than in one of primary irritant dermatitis.

CHAPTER 5

Erythemato-Squamous Eruptions

Psoriasis: Pityriasis Rosea: Seborrhoeic Dermatitis:
Lichen Planus: Exfoliative Dermatitis

The lesions of the following common dermatoses are characterized by redness and scaling. Lupus erythematosus and both tinea and syphilitic infections could be included under the heading of erythemato-squamous eruptions, but will be found elsewhere.

Psoriasis

This is a chronic and occasionally acute inflammatory disease, characterized by well-defined papules, or plaques of varying size (Figs. 10, 11; Plates 1, 2*). The lesions are reddish and covered with dull silvery scales.

It is found in people who are usually in good health, and is one of the commonest of all skin diseases.

CAUSE
Unknown.

Sex
It occurs equally in both sexes.

Age
Any age may be affected, and it may occur in infants a few months old. The commonest age is between 10 and 30.

Climate
It is commoner in northern climates and winter.

* All plates follow p. 148.

Heredity
The chance of contracting psoriasis is much greater if one or both parents or other ancestors have the disease, than if there is no relevant heredity. The familial incidence of all cases is about 30 per cent.

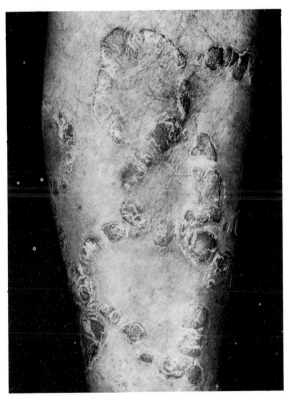

Fig. 10. Characteristic lesions on the front of the leg (Institute of Dermatology, University of London).

Predisposing factors

(1) Trauma, such as a laceration of the skin. (2) Acute infections, such as tonsillitis: this sort of history is not uncommon in children. (3) Psychological upsets.

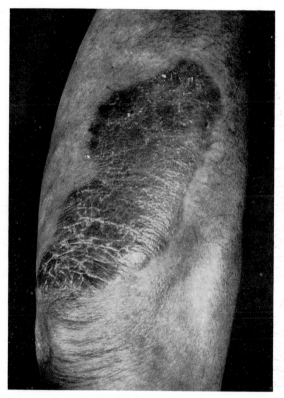

FIG. 11. Psoriasis.

PATHOLOGY

Parakeratosis is present, accounting for the clinically scaly appearance. Thinning of the upper areas of the papillae of the malpighian layer, with consequent lengthening of the rete pegs, results in blood vessels of the dermis lying closely adjacent to the parakeratotic area and altogether very much closer to the surface than in normal skin. When scales are forcibly removed, pin-point bleeding results because of the proximity of the blood vessels to the surface.

The dermis shows a mild or moderate inflammatory infiltrate.

CLINICAL FEATURES

There are usually no symptoms, apart from slight itching in rare cases. The onset as a rule is gradual, though occasionally explosive. The lesions are papular, dry and scaly. Their size is at first very small, even pin-point, and increases to various magnitudes; in some cases, a sheet of scales may cover half the trunk. Their shape is usually roughly circular, but many bizarre variations occur. The edges are always well defined. The surface is silvery and scaly, stopping short near the edge, where it is red. In early lesions, the scale is thin and

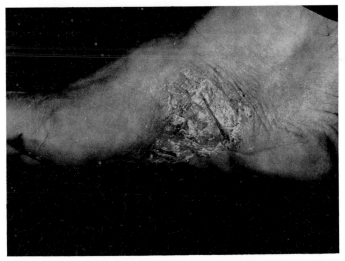

FIG. 12. Psoriasis. Simulating tinea and pompholyx (Institute of Dermatology, University of London).

as time passes the layer of scales thickens (Fig. 12). When scales are removed the underlying surface is shiny, red, and very smooth. Scrapings of this surface results in the development of pin-point haemorrhages (see Pathology). The red colour of the lesions becomes less vivid as they resolve.

Psoriasis characteristically attacks extensor surfaces, such as the

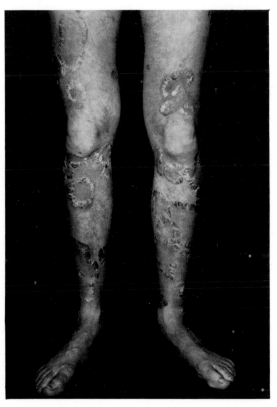

FIG. 13. Psoriasis. Characteristic situation (Institute of Dermatology, University of London).

knees and elbows, but any area may be involved (Fig. 13, Plate 3), and other favoured sites are scalp, sacral area, chest, face (Plate 4), abdomen, and genitalia. Scalp lesions are thick and round and better felt than seen. Under the palpating finger they are firm and the surface does not crumble as it would were the lesion crusted.

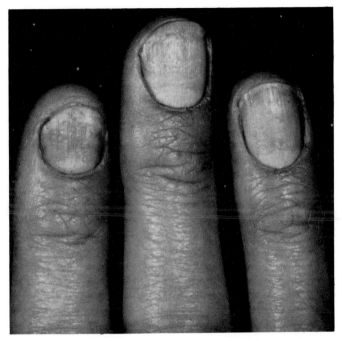

Fig. 14. Psoriasis. Thimble pitting (Institute of Dermatology, University of London).

The nail surfaces are attacked in about 30 per cent of cases following pitting, like that of a thimble (Fig. 14), and may be thickened at the free edge (Fig. 15). At the edge, a dirty brownish yellow staining may appear, elliptical or crescentic in shape, sometimes later involving the entire nail (Plate 5). Psoriasis may attack one nail or many, and in rare cases, nail involvement may be the only sign of the disease. Thimble-pitting is seen in other conditions, notably eczema.

Mucous membranes of the lips are very rarely involved.

The number of lesions varies from one or two to hundreds.

Special features

Koebner's phenomenon

This term is applied to lesions of psoriasis which develop at the site

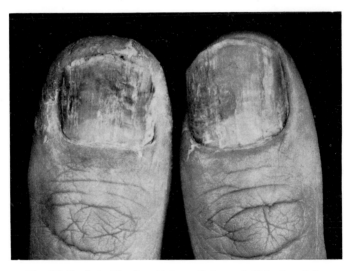

FIG. 15. Psoriasis. Showing ridging, splitting and thickening of the free edge of the nail (Institute of Dermatology, University of London).

of an injury, for example, a deep scratch being followed by psoriasis in the scratched area. It can only be produced when new lesions are appearing or old ones spreading. This phenomenon may also be seen in lichen planus, warts, and very occasionally in eczema.

COURSE

As the lesions start to clear, normal skin first appears in the centre, and in this state, to the untutored eye, can be confused with ringworm. Lastly, the residual margin clears. The course of the nail affection, which often resists all forms of treatment, is unpredictable.

Variations of psoriasis

1. Arthropathic: in this type severe polyarticular arthritis involving both small and large joints is found. By means of the Rose-Waaler differential sheep cell agglutination test, or various modifications of it, it is possible to differentiate the arthropathies; i.e. rheumatoid arthritis from most of the non-rheumatoid arthropathies and the pseudo-rheumatoid arthropathies.

2. Pustular: sterile firm pustules are found on the palms and soles with or without the usual psoriatic lesion elsewhere.

3. Erythrodermic or exfoliative: the most acute form of psoriasis, in which the entire skin is red and covered with fine scales, with the exception of a few diffusely-spread typical lesions.

Diagnostic aids

Biopsy.

DIAGNOSIS

This is made by the character of the lesion, and the involvement of the extensor surfaces.

For differential diagnosis see Table 1, p. 78.

TREATMENT

In no other condition, except eczema, is a more confident and optimistic approach required on the part of the doctor than in the management of this disease. Otherwise cure will be slow, and relapses common.

External

For chronic cases tar preparations are good for body lesions. The following regime is simple and not messy. (1) A daily bath (usually 100–125 litres of water) with 100 ml of liquor picis carbonis (tar) and 30–40 g of ung. emulsifications added to it; or Polytar emollient which is simpler to use. The patient lies in it for 10 minutes, and whilst immersed gently rubs off scales. (2) Later the same day the patient is exposed to ultra-violet rays (u.v.r.). (3) After u.v.r., Liq. Picis Carb. paint is applied to the lesions. Tar or dithranol ointment may be used in place of paint.

When this special regime is not used, a steroid cream should be applied, singly or in conjunction with polythene coverings (see p. 27).

The scalp lesions require tar ointments or steroid creams in conjunction with shampoos. Nail lesions resist treatment but sometimes clear up spontaneously. For acute cases, nothing but bland creams such as calamine or zinc should be used.

Internal

In acute psoriasis, and some cases of chronic psoriasis such as those resistant to topical treatment, the arthropathic cases, or those in which there is disabling psoriasis of the palms and soles, methotrexate and sometimes oral steroids are used. The former is the more effective. Its toxic effects are described on p. 35.

A single weekly dose of 25 mg at 1–2 week intervals is usually appropriate. If the response is inadequate, then the tablets are divided up into 3–4 doses to be given at 12-hour intervals. Methotrexate should not be used in patients below the age of puberty, in early pregnancy, or in alcoholics.

A more recent form of treatment is one in which methoxsalen tablets are given 2 hours before exposure to a high intensity UV A light source radiating at a continuous spectrum between 320 and 390 nm 3–4 days a week for 3–4 weeks. The treatment is known as PUVA (psoralen and UV A). Maintenance doses are then required for 12–24 weeks. No local treatment is necessary. Few adverse reactions have been noted to date, but it is not suitable for home treatment. Remissions of up to 18 months have been recorded.

For localized chronic lesions, intralesional injections of betamethasone-9-valerate, or triamcinolone are often effective.

PROGNOSIS

A permanent cure is impossible. Where there is a marked familial tendency, and/or a ready psoriatic response to emotional upsets, relapses are more likely. In general, the greater the faith of the patient in the doctor's handling of the disease, the longer are the periods of freedom from it.

Pityriasis Rosea

This is a mild inflammatory disease characterized by macules, and maculo-papular lesions, which are slightly scaly and formed mostly on the trunk (Fig. 16).

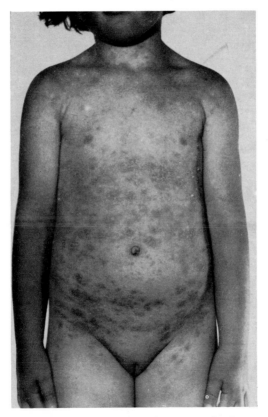

FIG. 16. Pityriasis rosea emphasizing the common involvement of trunk with scattered lesions on the arms and thighs (Department of Dermatology, Addenbrooke's Hospital).

CAUSE
Unknown.

Age
Appears at any age, but is commoner in young adults.

Season
Any time of year, but the period of highest incidence varies in
different parts of the world. In the U.K. it is commonest in the
autumn and winter months.

CLINICAL FEATURES
Symptoms
Usually there are no symptoms, but sometimes there is headache and
malaise, or itching. Onset is sudden, heralded by the appearance of a
solitary macular lesion. This first lesion is known as the 'herald patch'
and there is an interval of a week or ten days before other lesions
appear, while the 'herald patch' persists alone. If it appears on the

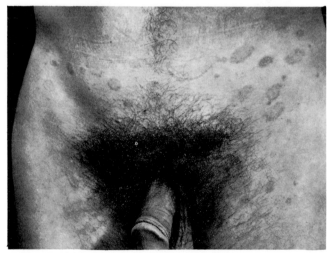

FIG. 17. Pityriasis rosea. Superficial, maculo-papular, slightly scaly
lesions (Institute of Dermatology, University of London).

back, it may not be noticed by the patient. Very occasionally it fails to appear.

Lesions are macular, some are slightly raised becoming maculo-papular (Fig. 17). The size varies from pin-head to penny size or larger. Their shape tends to be oval, with the long axis running along the lines of cleavage of the skin, so that a streamlining effect is noticed. The edges are quite well defined. The surface is always scaly. In early lesions, the scale is restricted to the centre, the actual edges being free of scale, and later the scale breaks, leaving a gap in the centre. In older lesions, the scale is markedly at the edge, scalloped and forming a delicate collarette (Fig. 18). The colour is rose or red (Plate 6). The sites are characteristically the trunk and upper half of the arms and legs. Only occasionally are the lower halves of the limbs, the palms, face, and scalp involved, and then most commonly in children. The number of lesions varies from several to hundreds.

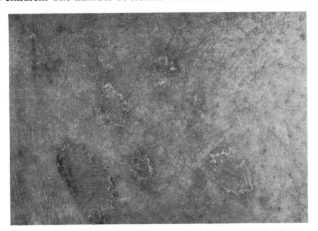

Fig. 18. Pityriasis rosea. Close-up of lesions showing typical collarette of scales (Department of Dermatology, Addenbrooke's Hospital).

COURSE

A week or so after the 'herald patch', many lesions appear and multiply for two or three weeks. Resolution then occurs within six to ten weeks of the onset.

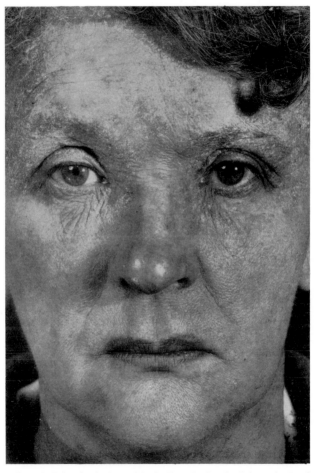

Fig. 19. Seborrhoeic dermatitis. Scaling also involved the scalp (Institute of Dermatology, University of London).

DIAGNOSIS

By the character and distribution of the lesions. For differential diagnosis see p. 78.

TREATMENT

Calamine lotion may be required to suppress itching in a few cases. The patient should be told that the disease is not infectious, the prognosis is good, and that it will disappear in 6–8 weeks.

PROGNOSIS

This is excellent. Relapses and second attacks are very uncommon.

Seborrhoeic Dermatitis

This is an acute, subacute, or chronic inflammatory scaly disease of hairy areas, well endowed with sebaceous glands (Fig. 19). Seborrhoeic dermatitis of the scalp is basically an increase in the normal amount of scaling of the epidermis, which is known as *dandruff* or *pityriasis capitis* (pityron-bran), superimposed by inflammation. Seborrhoea may or may not be present. Other areas attacked by seborrhoeic dermatitis in a similar fashion are the axillae, sub-mammary folds, umbilicus, groins and natal cleft. The cause is unknown.

CLINICAL FEATURES

The onset is gradual. The lesions are macular or papular, pin-head to sixpenny size, rounded, and greyish or dirty yellow in colour (Fig. 20). The surface consists of greasy scales, some of which can be rubbed off. When the external ear is involved it becomes crusted and may show fissuring at the back. Blepharitis may be present. When the other areas mentioned above are affected, the lesions are similar to those on the scalp.

The condition may be complicated by *eczematization*, when the lesions suddenly produce a sero-purulent exudate.

DIAGNOSIS

This is made by the character of the lesions involving seborrhoeic areas. Differential diagnosis is described on page 78.

TREATMENT

Scalp. Shampoos should be given daily until the head is free from crusts; and then twice weekly. Genisol and Polytar shampoos are useful. For severe cases, Alphosyl cream (contains coal tar extract) or ung. picis co. should be applied daily, for less severe ones, salicylic acid lotion B.P.C. When eczematization has developed, as evidenced by extensive oozing and crusting, applications of a steroid

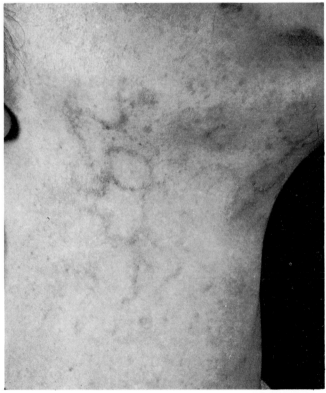

FIG. 20. Seborrhoeic dermatitis. Polycyclic lesions, suggesting tinea (Institute of Dermatology, University of London).

lotion combined with an antibiotic should be made two or three times a day, until the intense inflammation has subsided, before applying creams or lotions.

Face and Ears. A steroid lotion with or without an antibiotic is usually effective. If it fails, recourse should be made to Salicylic acid ointment B.P. with 2 per cent sulph. ppt.

Body. Treatment as for the face.

PROGNOSIS

Generally good, although recurrences are not uncommon, especially as regards scalp lesions. For the scalp, therefore, it is advisable to apply the lotion advised above periodically, and to shampoo the scalp regularly. The immediate outlook in acute cases is more favourable when over-zealous treatment is avoided.

Lichen Planus

This is an acute or chronic inflammatory disease, characterized by papules which are flat-topped, polygonal, shiny, violaceous and slightly scaly, found chiefly on the flexor surfaces (Plates 7 and 8). The mucous membranes are commonly involved. Itching of the skin is usual and may be quite severe.

CAUSE

This is unknown.

Sex

Women are more affected than men.

Age

Adults are most commonly affected, although no age after 10 is exempt.

Predisposing factors: 1. Psychological upsets often precede an attack. 2. Trauma. A scratch or more serious injury sometimes produces the first lesion.

PATHOLOGY

Hyperkeratosis, increase of the granular layer, irregular acanthosis often showing a saw-tooth appearance, and destruction of the basal layer by a band-like infiltrate, which hugs the epidermis. Oral lesions show a similar picture.

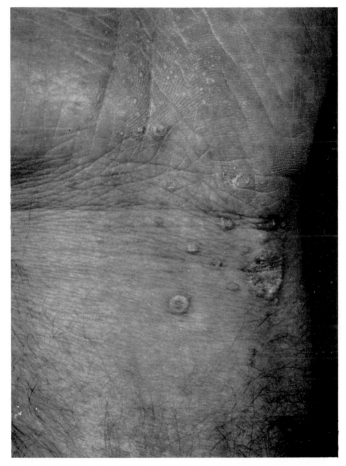

FIG. 21. Lichen planus. Polygonal scaly papules on the wrist and palm, with one annular lesion (Institute of Dermatology, University of London).

CLINICAL FEATURES

Itching may be slight or severe, and is usually intermittent. The onset is sudden or gradual. Lesions are papular, dry and slightly scaly. Their shape on close examination is polymorphic and polygonal (Fig. 21, Plate 9). Their size is at first pin-point, and increases up to pea-size. Later, neighbouring lesions may join, forming large patches of varying shapes. The surface of many small lesions is dimpled, and all lesions are scaly; the scale in some may be very thin and adherent, making it difficult to observe, but gentle friction will demonstrate it. Shininess of the surface is a diagnostic feature, but the lesion may have to be examined from different aspects in good light to reveal this sign.

The colour is essentially red at first, altering in several weeks to violaceous and as the disease clears, to dull brownish. The density of these colours is often interrupted by fine milky-looking streaks and dots, especially in the early phase. They are known as Wickham's striae, and are useful aids to diagnosis.

Sites most commonly attacked are the front of the wrists, the thighs, waist and penis. Lesions are seldom found on the scalp, face, palms or soles. Mucous membranes are affected in 25–70 per cent of all cases. The lesions on the inner sides of the cheeks are tiny milky-white papules, or are arranged in a network pattern of thin thread-like streaks. The lips, tongue (Plate 10), and palate may be similarly affected.

The nails are affected in about 10 per cent of cases, and in some patients, the nails may be affected without skin lesions being present. The nail changes are non-specific and may appear as longitudinal furrows, which vary in depth, with normal nail-plate forming ridges; there may be uniform thinning of the nail-plate; or shedding of one or several nails. The loss may or may not be permanent, depending on the degree of matrix involvement.

Special features

Koebner's phenomenon is common (see psoriasis).

Some other clinical varieties

(1) Lichen planus hypertrophicus. In this type the lesions are much thicker than in the common variety and at first glance seem to be warty. They are usually found exclusively on the fronts of the legs.

There is no dimpling and shininess is not obvious. At the edge of these hypertrophic lesions (Plate 11), the typical flat-topped, polygonal, polymorphic papules of lichen planus may be found. Itching is present.

(2) Lichen planus bullosus. In this variety, vesicles and bullae appear during the course of the disease.

Diagnostic aids
Biopsy.

DIAGNOSIS
By character of lesions. For differential diagnosis see page 78.

TREATMENT
Attention should be paid to the general health of the patient, especially with regard to any emotional stresses that exist, but treatment does not seem to have much effect on the course of the disease.

External
Steroid creams used singly or in conjunction with polythene coverings (see page 27). Betamethasone pellets 0·1 mg t.d.s. often benefit oral lesions. Superficial X-rays and grenz rays are useful for the hypertrophic variety of skin lesions, when all else fails.

Internal
Steroids are beneficial in acute cases and often in the hypertrophic variety, where intra-lesional steroid injections may be used.

PROGNOSIS
This condition usually lasts six months to two years. Relapses may sometimes occur after apparent cure.

Exfoliative Dermatitis

This condition is characterized by generalized scaling and redness. It is usually a complication of a pre-existing skin disease, or drug intoxication. It may very rarely appear primarily, by itself.

CAUSE

Age
It is most common in middle life.

Sex
More common in males than females, the proportion being about three to one.

Predisposing factors
Psoriasis. Eczema. Seborrhoeic dermatitis. Reticuloses, such as leukaemia, or Hodgkin's disease. Drug intoxications such as arsenic (administered orally, by injection, or as vaginal pessaries), sulphonamides, penicillin.

CLINICAL FEATURES

A constant feeling of being cold, associated with shivering and fever, is characteristic. Itching is variable, and may be intense.

The onset is gradual. Lesions are macular. Their size is at first coin to palm-size, but soon lesions coalesce to form large patches until there is little or no normal skin to be seen. The surface is covered with small thin scales, or large sheets of scales. Occasionally an uneven yellowish exudate may appear. The entire skin surface becomes very red. The sites involved may be anywhere on the body. The scalp lesions become matted and crusted. The hair loses its normal lustre, becomes brittle, and falls, so that thinning is noticeable. The nails cease growing normally, are dull in appearance and in severe cases may be shed.

COURSE

This varies, and waxing and waning of lesions is characteristic. Recurrences are common, although treatment by steroids has reduced their frequency.

DIAGNOSIS

This is made by the redness of the skin, the diffuse scaling, and constitutional symptoms. It must be differentiated from psoriasis. The essential diagnosis is the condition underlying the exfoliative dermatitis.

TREATMENT

Rest in bed, with particular attention to the avoidance of bedsores which are most likely to occur in the elderly patient. A high protein diet should be maintained.

TABLE 1

Differential diagnosis of the commonest scaly conditions

	Character of scale	Distribution	Itching	Onset
Eczema-Dermatitis	Dry, fragmented covered lesion	Any	Present	Variable
Psoriasis	Dry, silvery when scratched; do not reach periphery of lesion	Extensors	Absent	Gradual
Seborrhoeic Dermatitis	Dry or greasy, greyish or dirty-yellow	Hairy areas and creases	Absent	Insidious
Pityriasis Rosea	Dry, broken in centre of lesion, forms a frill at edge	Trunk	Uncommon	Sudden
Tinea	Dry, peripheral. Some residual scales may remain in centre of lesion	Any	Slight	Sudden or gradual depending on type of fungus present
Lichen planus	Adherent, and thin	Flexors	Present	Sudden or gradual
Lupus erythematosus	Adherent, with plugging of follicles by scales	Face, scalp, ears. Rarely elsewhere	Absent	Gradual

External

Oatmeal baths daily, provided the patient is fit enough to endure them. A bland greasy application such as Oily Cream B.P.C. or Thovaline cream is useful. Drying lotions or sprays should not be used.

Internal

Steroids are particularly beneficial in these cases. Treatment of the underlying condition must be kept in mind.

PROGNOSIS

This depends to some extent on the nature of the primary condition. Recurrences and relapses should be carefully watched for in exfoliative dermatitis.

CHAPTER 6

Erythematous Eruptions

Toxic Erythema: Erythema multiforme: Erythema nodosum:
Urticaria: Rosacea

The conditions described in this chapter are all mainly characterized by erythema. Erythema is a redness which fades on pressure but which returns rapidly on its release.

Toxic Erythema

The cause is usually hypersensitivity to such foods as shell-fish, mushrooms, or strawberries; or drugs such as penicillin or barbiturates; or to external causes, e.g. trusses or splints.

The eruptions are generally bilateral and symmetrical, affecting the trunk, face and upper parts of the limbs. They are usually morbilliform, or scarlatiniform. General malaise and slight pyrexia are present and the attack clears up in a week or so.

DIAGNOSIS

This is made from specific fevers rather than pyrexias of unknown origin. Drug eruptions should also be considered.

TREATMENT

The cause is treated if found. Otherwise simple measures such as a Calamine lotion suffice.

Erythema Multiforme

This is an acute inflammatory condition characterized by macules, papules, vesicles and sometimes bullae, symmetrically distributed.

Generally, it should be considered as a toxic eruption.

CAUSE

In many cases this is undiscovered but considered to be possibly viral. Where the disease is of this type it is commoner in spring and autumn, and occurs in children.

In other cases, it may be secondary to the following conditions:

(i) Drug intoxication—antibiotics such as sulphonamides and penicillin, quinine, salicylates.

(ii) Systemic diseases, such as glandular or rheumatic fever, pneumonia, nephritis or meningitis.

(iii) Serum sickness, following the injection of antitoxins.

(iv) Pregnancy is sometimes accompanied by it between the 5th and 7th month; the eruption fades early in the post-natal period.

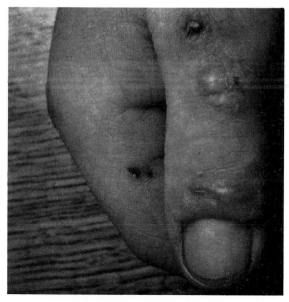

FIG. 22. Erythema multiforme. Bullous lesions.

PATHOLOGY

The blood vessels are dilated, surrounded by cellular infiltration. When vesicles or bullae are present, they are uni- or multilocular, and sub-epidermal. Acantholysis is absent.

CLINICAL FEATURES

In most cases there is a prodromal phase of malaise; in severe cases, sore throat, diarrhoea, and pyrexia. In some cases, no symptoms occur.

The onset is sudden. Lesions are macular and papular. Their size varies from pin-point to pea-size; later coalescence of the lesions may occur. Their shape is round, the centre being darker than the rest of the lesion, like the iris of the eye (Fig. 22, Plate 12). The colour is red, but always disappears on pressure.

Backs of the hands and forearms are the sites most commonly attacked. The sides of the neck, the face and legs, genitalia, and in 50 per cent of cases the mucous membranes may also be involved.

COURSE

The disease usually lasts 3–4 weeks.

OTHER VARIETIES

The Stevens-Johnson Syndrome
is also known by the more descriptive term of erythema bullosum malignans. It is similar to erythema multiforme, but the clinical features are far more severe, the most marked ones being high fever, widespread and painful involvement of the mucous membranes and joint pains. This condition may be fatal.

DIAGNOSIS

This is made by the redness of the lesions, the iris lesions when present, the bilateral distribution, and the absence of itching.

Urticaria presents itchy weals and these are rarely symmetrical. When vesicles or bullae are present, *pemphigus* has to be excluded. The bullae of pemphigus arise from normal skin, those of this condition from red macules. *Dermatitis herpetiformis* is an itchy vesicular or bullous eruption. Drug eruptions, toxic erythemas and pemphigoid may have to be considered.

TREATMENT

Causes if known, must be treated. Rest in bed is essential in severe and preferable in moderate cases.

External

Eusol lotion or aluminium acetate 5 per cent lotion may help.

Internal

Oxytetracyclines by mouth may be required to suppress secondary infection. In severe cases, and especially in the Stevens-Johnson syndrome, steroids are indicated, involving initial daily doses of 30–40 mg or more of prednisolone.

PROGNOSIS

Mild and moderate cases are liable to recur once a year for a few years.

Erythema Nodosum

This is an acute inflammatory condition characterized by painful nodules usually on the fronts of the legs (Plate 13), but occasionally on the outer sides of the forearms. It is *symptomatic* of a bacterial, viral or fungal disease, a drug eruption, or a concomitant condition. Streptococcal conditions are probably the commonest cause.

CAUSE

Age

It occurs commonly between 20 and 30 years.

Sex

Females are more affected than males.

Seasons

It occurs more commonly in the first half of the year.

Associated conditions

Streptococcal, as noted above. Sarcoidosis, rheumatic fever, tinea, tuberculosis, syphilis, leprosy, and certain rare viral diseases. Drugs may be responsible, including the contraceptive pill.

PATHOLOGY

There is a heavy infiltrate in and around the vessels of the dermis, with a few lymphocytes and plasma cells. The infiltrate is also found in the subcutaneous fat. Streptococci or other bacteria may be seen.

CLINICAL FEATURES

The onset is acute, with malaise, fever, and some joint pains. The lesions are nodular, being painful, red and shiny. They reach their full size, about 2–5 cm in diameter, in 24 hours and last about two weeks, healing without scarring. The lesions appear in crops in a characteristic fashion.

DIAGNOSIS

This is made by the symmetry and tenderness of the lesions. The condition must be distinguished from erythema induratum (Plate 14), which occurs on the calves of the legs, rarely in crops, and tends to ulcerate.

TREATMENT

The cause must be sought, and treated. Cool aluminium acetate compresses are soothing.

PROGNOSIS

The disease lasts about 3–4 weeks, and rarely recurs.

Urticaria

This is an acute, chronic or recurrent disorder, characterized by transient weals and papules (Fig. 23), accompanied by itching and pricking sensations. It is also known as nettle-rash.

CAUSE

This is often very difficult to find and, in 50 per cent of cases, remains undiscovered. Some cases, but by no means all, are caused by an immune reaction. The pharmacological agents which cause urticaria can be released in other ways, such as injury or cold. Four of these have so far been identified: (1) histamine; (2) slow reacting substance A; (3) serotonin (5H-T); and the so-called plasma kinins.

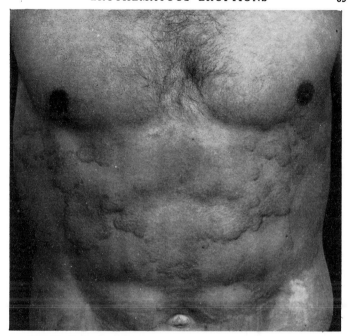

FIG. 23. Urticaria showing papules and weals (Institute of Dermatology, University of London).

Sex
Women are more affected than men, especially in the case of chronic urticaria.

Age
Any age may be affected, but it is commoner in the third and fourth decades.

Allergy (*see* p. 11)
This is the commonest cause of urticaria. Many different substances may be included under this heading:

(i)   Foods: e.g. shell-fish, strawberries, pork, eggs.
(ii) Drugs: penicillin, aspirin, enemas, codeine and others.
(iii) Parasites: fleas, lice, intestinal worms.
(iv) Physical agents: heat, cold, pressure.
(v)   Inhalants: house dust, feathers.

Psychogenic
This group accounts for quite a large proportion of cases of chronic
urticaria, anxiety neuroses and emotional conflicts commonly being
responsible. Psychological stress, however, is a part of everyone's
daily experience and care must be taken for this reason both to
consider it as a cause and to avoid too ready a tendency to give it
sole blame.

PATHOLOGY
Vascular dilatation occurs in the dermal vessels, with an outpouring
of serum and white cells. This collection of fluid compresses the
vessels, so that there may be blanching at the centre of the weal.
As the fluid increases, it makes its way through the epidermis to
produce a vesicle, or bulla. These phenomena occur as a result of
liberation of histamine in the skin.

CLINICAL FEATURES
The onset is sudden. Itching is present to a variable degree. The
weals last for a few hours, and not more than 48 hours. The weals of
physical urticaria clear within an hour. Their size lies between that
of a pea to palm size or larger. Their shape also varies and may be
very irregular when coalescence of lesions occurs. The surface may
be smooth, vesicular or bullous, and they are red, although central
blanching may occur. The number may be few or many. Any area
may be involved, but arms, legs, thighs and waist are the most
favoured. The mucous membranes are also commonly attacked,
especially the larynx.

Special features
Dermographism may be noted in urticaria (Fig. 24), and is characterized by the ease with which weals are provoked by rubbing the
skin with a blunt instrument. But it is also found in 5 per cent of the
normal population.

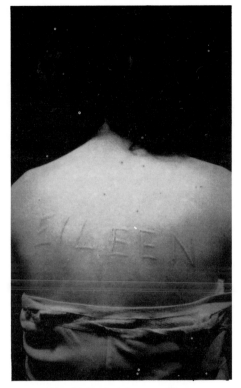

FIG. 24. Typical dermographism.

Laboratory findings
Eosinophilia is common, but inconstant. The total lymphocytes may be reduced in chronic urticaria.

COURSE

Acute urticaria clears up in a few days or weeks; chronic urticaria may persist for weeks, months or years.

Other clinical varieties
(i) Bullous, often seen in children. (ii) Giant urticaria, or angio-neurotic oedema, which differs from ordinary urticaria only in the size of the lesions. In this type, the eyelids, lips, the lobes of the ears and genitalia are most commonly involved. When the eyelids are affected the patient may find it nearly impossible to see, and lip lesions may affect eating. Transient attacks of colicky pain are frequent.

DIAGNOSIS
This is made by the presence of transient weals whose duration does not exceed 48 hours. *Scabies* must be excluded, by a search for burrows.

TREATMENT
Prophylactic
If the cause can be discovered, it must be avoided; it is usually food or a drug.

External
Calamine, steroid lotions and sprays are palliative.

Internal
Many anti-histamines are effective and are given in liquid form to children, in tablet form to adults. For adults, chlorpheniramine maleate (Piriton) 4 mg t.d.s., or triprolidine (Actidil) 2·5 mg t.d.s. may be given. Sometimes a double dose may be required. For children these doses are graduated according to age.
   Oral steroids may have to be given for severe and chronic cases after considerable thought. There is no doubt, however, that they are helpful.

PROGNOSIS
This is difficult to assess as improvement often occurs without a specific cause or treatment being determined.

Rosacea

This is a chronic inflammatory disorder involving the central area of the face, usually seen with acneiform lesions and telangiectases.

CAUSE

This is not exactly known, but anything giving rise to persistent reflex flushing of the face provokes its development.

Sex

Far more common in women.

Age

From the age of 30 and in women most noticeably at or about the menopause.

Predisposing Factors

Occupation. Those exposed to a great deal of sunlight or severe winds, such as farmers and sailors, are prone to attacks.

Food. Chronic alcoholism and a spicy diet may aggravate rosacea.

Psychological. Patients are usually depressed, but the depression is probably due to their facial disfigurement.

PATHOLOGY

There is dilatation and the formation of new capillaries which account for the redness of the lesions. There is also a dermal lympho-cytic infiltrate, which sometimes gives the lesions a rather brownish colour. The sebaceous glands are occasionally hypertrophied, which produces rhinophyma (see below).

CLINICAL FEATURES

The onset is gradual, with bouts of facial flushing usually being the first symptom. Lesions may be papular and pustular, although redness usually predominates. The chin, cheeks, nose and forehead may be involved, severally or singly and occasionally the neck and chest also. The cheeks and nose are known as the butterfly area of the face (Plate 15). In this acneiform condition there are no blackheads.

Other varieties

Rhinophyma may develop. This gross hypertrophy of the nose is associated with easily visible pitting and marked redness. It is commonest in men, and alcoholics.

Complications
Conjunctivitis, iritis and keratitis occasionally occur. These signs in some cases precede the onset of the facial lesions, but usually follow them.

DIAGNOSIS

This is made by the distribution on the butterfly area of the face and the absence of blackheads. *Acne vulgaris* always presents comedones (blackheads), and involves any area of the face, as well as the chest and back. *Lupus erythematosus* appears as well-defined patches on the face, without acneiform lesions.

TREATMENT

Predisposing factors must be avoided as much as possible. Rest periods should be increased and regularly taken.

External
A steroid lotion is nearly always helpful, but if it is not, 1 per cent sulphur in calamine lotion may be tried. Long continued use of steroid lotions, e.g. betamethasone (Betnovate) on the face can produce undesirable side effects such as atrophy and telangiectases, and thus, their use is restricted.

Gentle daily massage with cold cream, from the centre of the face outwards, performed at night, is often surprisingly beneficial.

Internal
Oxytetracyclines when taken for long periods, as for acne vulgaris, produce good results. Antacids before meals are indicated, if symptoms of dyspepsia are present.

Rhinophyma is treated by plastic surgery.

PROGNOSIS

Mild cases usually respond rapidly to treatment, but in others relapses are disappointingly frequent.

CHAPTER 7

Diseases due to Physical or Chemical Substances

Drug Eruptions: Sunburn: Prickly Heat: Chilblains: Bed Sores

Drug Eruptions

There is no categorical method of describing the appearance of a drug eruption, as it may imitate some features of practically any other disease. It is, however, the bizarre tendency to produce some but not all features of another disease which should make one consider this diagnosis as a possibility.

Such eruptions are caused by drugs ingested, injected, or otherwise absorbed and should not be confused with eruptions caused by external applications.

CAUSE

Little is known about the exact way in which drugs cause eruptions, but certain theories are accepted.

Allergy seems to produce some reactions, but there are no skin tests to prove it.

Idiosyncrasy in some people leads to the appearance of an eruption and may result from sensitivity to a drug which had previously caused dermatitis through topical application. The dermatitis, a thing of the past, may have been forgotten by the patient. This thing of the past, may have been forgotten by the patient. Idiosyncracy applies especially to sulphonamide and penicillin ointments, which are now never used by dermatologists.

Overdosage, either self-inflicted or unintentionally, or by accidental errors in the pharmacy. Imapired renal excretion may also result in reduced excretion of the drug.

Genetic factors sometimes determine an individual's reaction to a drug.

Any *age* may be affected, females more than males, and anxiety-prone individuals are more susceptible.

CLINICAL FEATURES

The onset varies with the drug concerned, from sudden (e.g. penicillin) to attenuated (e.g. barbiturates). The lesions may be urticarial, erythematous, vesicular, bullous, purpuric or pustular.

Distribution is generalized, except in the fixed drug eruption (see below). The colour is often curiously bright. In the case of some drug eruptions the lesions are characteristic and these will be specifically described below. A great many are non-specific and will be grouped under one heading (see below).

DIAGNOSIS

In some cases, the diagnosis can be made at a glance. Typically, the onset is sudden, the rash widespread, bright and symmetrical and the history coincides with the taking of a drug. In other cases the diagnosis must be considered when the eruption is either distinctly peculiar and does not fit into any known pattern of disease, or is bullous, or is present as an exfoliative dermatitis.

Having considered the possibility of a drug eruption, it is important to know which common drugs may be associated with the presenting skin reaction and, conversely, to know the peculiar and unique presentations of a few drugs in common use.

A. ERUPTIONS, AND SOME DRUGS WHICH PRODUCE THEM

1. *Urticaria*. Penicillin, isoniazid, salicylates.

2. *Morbilliform and scarlatiniform*. Penicillin, sulphonamides, chloramphenicol, phenylbutazone, barbiturates, anti-histamines.

3. *Vesicular and bullous*. Iodides, bromides, sulphonamides, dapsone.

4. *Purpura*. Salicylates, carbromal, chloramphenicol. An itchy rash develops, especially on the buttocks and legs.

5. *Light-sensitivity eruptions*. Sulphonamides, phenothiazine tranquillizers. The rash is limited to exposed areas.

6. *Exfoliative dermatitis*. Gold and all heavy metals.

7. *Fixed drug eruption.* Phenolphthalein (in laxatives), antipyrine, and barbiturates.

The lesion is well circumscribed, dusky red, and usually on the trunk, or upper parts of the limbs. It lasts a few days and leaves a hyperpigmented patch. There may be one or more patches and they always reappear in the same site, following the taking of the drug.

8. *Lichenoid.* Anti-malarials, gold, bismuth, amiphenazole, phenothiazine.

B. SOME DRUGS, AND THEIR TYPE OF ERUPTION

Aspirin may cause urticaria and even when it is not the cause, it should be withheld, as it may arrest recovery.

Arsenic, as liquor arsenicalis (Fowler's solution) given over a long period may give rise to pigmentation, keratotic lesions of the palms and soles, and eventually intra-epidermal carcinomata. While it is now rarely used, it is still the occasional ingredient of some tonics, and solutions used by agricultural and vineyard workers.

Antibiotics of the broad-spectrum variety, e.g. tetracyclines, may produce ano-genital pruritus.

Barbiturates may cause urticarial, erythematous, purpuric, bullous, and fixed eruptions. Aphthae and stomatitis also occur.

Bromides and iodides may cause an acneiform eruption, but without the blackheads, which occur in true acne. Infants may suffer by transmission of the drug through the mother's milk.

Chloroquine (Nivaquine) may cause difficulty with focusing, photophobia, and retinopathy after prolonged courses, as well as permanent and progressive retinal damage, although the changes may be reversible in the early stages.

Chlorpromazine (Largactil) may produce various erythemata, with light sensitivity an added factor, and lichenoid eruptions (Fig. 25). Cross-reactions with related drugs prescribed as tranquillizers, or antihistamines, may occur.

Penicillin. Urticaria is the commonest eruption which may be chronic and severe. Sensitization and subsequent eruptions in babies may occur through the drinking of a mother's or a cow's milk, if they have been given penicillin. Penicillin is the most common cause of drug eruptions.

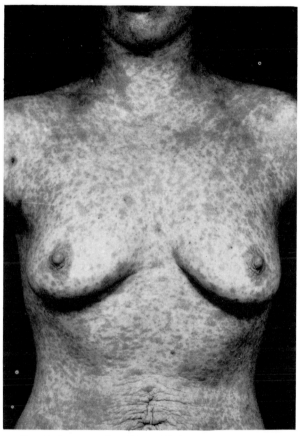

Fig. 25. Drug eruption: lichenoid lesions due to chloroquine.

Serum can cause urticaria or erythema, one or two weeks after injection.

Steroids may produce hirsuties, hyperpigmentation and acneiform eruptions.

TREATMENT

Most drug eruptions clear up within a week of stopping the drug. The taking of the smallest amount of the drug will result in a relapse. Plenty of fluids should be given to hasten elimination of the drug.

Antihistamines, e.g. triprolidine (Actidil) 2·5 mg or chlorpheniramine maleate (Piriton) 4 mg three times a day are useful in the early phase of penicillin urticaria. They are obviously contraindicated in chlorpromazine eruptions.

The management of each drug eruption cannot be briefly dealt with here.

Sunburn

This is caused by ultra-violet rays from the sun. First or second degree burns may follow a few hours of exposure, blondes being more sensitive than brunettes.

Severe sunburn is treated in the same way as thermal burns, with local and/or systemic steroids. Indomethicin may also be useful. Calamine cream is effective in mild cases. For prophylaxis, isoamyl-p-N, N-dimethylaminobenzoate 2·5 per cent (Spectraban lotion), or Mexenone 4 per cent cream (Uvistat) will partially protect the skin.

Prickly Heat

Miliaria

This condition is characterized by pin-point to pin-head sized vesicles and papules, accompanied by prickling and burning sensations, and is due to inflammation of sweat ducts.

It is a feature of tropical life, or work which entails exposure to excessive heat.

TREATMENT

Light clothing should be worn. Heavy meals and alcohol must be avoided. Cool bran or oatmeal baths are useful. Steroid sprays are temporarily beneficial. High doses of vitamin C may help.

PROGNOSIS

Once the tendency to prickly heat is established, it can rarely be abolished.

Chilblains

Perniosis

This painful condition is characterized by itchy, red or nodular lesions on the fingers, toes, ears or face which occasionally ulcerate. They result from hyperactivity of the peripheral vessels in response to cold and they are most common in young women and children.

They may be mistaken for erythema induratum (p. 121) or erythema nodosum (p. 83).

TREATMENT

Warm clothing is essential; cold must be avoided. Toilet lanoline applied in the morning may act as a partial insulator.

A strong erythema dose of irradiation from an ultra-violet radiation lamp, once a week for three successive weeks, in September and October, may protect the treated areas for the ensuing winter (Ingram).

Bedsores

A bedsore is a sore caused by lying in bed, or sitting in a chair, due solely to pressure. Tissue damage due to local ischaemia occurs from pressure. Most bedsores develop during the course of an illness, in old people.

TREATMENT

This usually consists of (1) local and systemic antibiotics, (2) control of pressure, (3) transfusions, (4) high calorie and protein diet, (5) steroids by mouth, (6) physio- and occupational therapy, (7) surgical methods when necessary.

Prophylactic treatment entails the use of such aids as ripple beds, regular turning every 2–4 hours although patients dislike it, and keeping the skin dry and clean, with Talc Dusting Powder B.P.C. or Zinc Starch + Talc Dusting Powder (B.P.C.). Avoid surgical spirit as it cracks the skin.

CHAPTER 8

Psychological Factors in Skin Diseases

Pruritus: Senile Pruritus: Ano-Genital Pruritus:
Dermatitis Artefacta: Trichotillomania:
Neurotic Excoriations

Introduction

The awareness of the relationship between the skin and the mind, in health and disease, has been evident in literature for the past 2,000 years. To-day, expressions such as 'becoming hot under the collar', 'rubbing the skin up the wrong way', or 'someone getting under one's skin' are the modern reflection of this association and of cutaneous reactions to shame, guilt, anger and anxiety.

Nothing actually happens in our minds without affecting our bodies and the reverse is also true, body and mind referring only to two different aspects of the single indivisible whole. When our body or mind is not precariously poised in a critical incident, the relationship between them is scarcely noticed. But when shame, guilt, or anxiety, for example, introduce a disturbance into the interaction of the body and mind, physical reactions occur which vary from those recognizable by the man-in-the-street, to those whose significance is often variously calculated by differing physicians. Those readily recognizable are an increased pulse rate, vague precordial pain, indigestion or sweating, then physicians have to assess the relationship of these heart, stomach or skin symptoms and signs.

There are some apparently substantial reasons for the skin being affected by emotional disturbances. It is obviously used for expression, as blushing or pallor show. It has more pathways leading to the brain than any other organ, and is therefore closely associated with fundamental emotional deviations. The skin is also used in daily life for the reinforcement of confidence by means of beautification and dress.

97

However, very few skin diseases are a DIRECT result of psychological disorders.

They are:

1. Dermatitis artefacta.
2. Trichotillomania.
3. Parasitophobia and other phobias.
4. Neurotic excoriations.

There are, however, many skin diseases which are sometimes triggered off by emotional upsets, but are not directly attributable to them.

Amongst this group are:

1. Allergic conditions.
2. Alopecia areata.
3. Pompholyx.
4. Eczema—dermatitis (hay-fever—asthma syndrome).
5. Hyperidrosis.
6. Localized neurodermatitis.
7. Ano-genital pruritus.
8. Psoriasis.
9. Rosacea.
10. Urticaria.

When investigating a case for emotional factors, and then discovering them, the tendency to lose sight of causal somatic factors is considerable. It is therefore more than ever important first to exclude organic causes. The cases in which organic sources are missed as factors in the cause of skin disease greatly outnumber those in which psychological factors are missed, for the reason mentioned above. In many instances, it is important not to be misled by the patient's conception of the onset of the disease, which seems so felicitously to suit the case. When psychological factors appear to be the pivot around which the cause revolves, the results of psychotherapy are extremely difficult to evaluate, since they are invariably associated with simultaneous topical treatment. It seems therefore that the role of psychotherapy in this group is essentially supportive rather than leading.

Except for the following types of pruritus, the conditions named above have been dealt with elsewhere.

Pruritus

Pruritus is itching, which may be generalized or localized. Pruritus is considered to be due to the stimulation of the subepidermal nerve plexuses, by proteolytic enzymes, which are released from the epidermis as a result of either primary irritation, or allergic sensitization reactions.

Pruritus may occur without any cutaneous lesions, in conditions such as Hodgkin's disease, pregnancy, diabetes mellitus, thyrotoxicosis, or senile skin. The greatest number of such cases are due to psychological causes, and it is these factors which should be carefully investigated.

Senile Pruritus

This is probably due to ischaemic and atrophic skin changes. Itching is spasmodic and often mercilessly severe.

TREATMENT

This is usually disappointing. Local treatment such as steroid sprays provide only temporary relief. Sedatives such as phenobarbitone, 100 mg three times a day, may help. In severe cases it is necessary to give steroids by mouth. Prednisolone, 5 mg three times a day, often produces the greatest respite from itching; after two or three weeks it may be reduced to a minimal dosage of 5 or 2·5 mg daily and eventually stopped altogether.

Ano-Genital Pruritus

Pruritus vulvae, ani, or scroti

Organic causes which must be excluded before psychological factors can be considered are:

1. Diabetes.
2. Vaginal infections, such as trichomonas vaginalis.
3. Urinary infections.
4. Threadworm infestations, in children.

These can be easily excluded.

Other less usual conditions are:

5. Contact dermatitis from contraceptive sheaths or pessaries.
6. Ringworm or candidiasis.
7. Seborrhoeic dermatitis.
8. Psoriasis.
9. Antibiotics taken orally, especially tetracyclines.
10. Lice.
11. Menopausal atrophy.

Elimination of these conditions justifies the taking of a history in search of psychological causes.

The cause may be a superficial one easy to deal with, such as a passing anxiety. More often, however, the problems are deep and complicated, involving perhaps a revolt against intercourse, for reasons of incompatible appetites, fear of pregnancy, or the presence of a third party.

In these cases psychotherapy may be invaluable, but must still be accompanied by local treatment, the best of which is in the form of a steroid lotion or cream.

Recurrences are not unusual, and the management depends to a great extent on the confidence of the physician and the patient's acceptance of it.

Localized Neurodermatitis

Lichen simplex chronicus

This is a chronic low-grade inflammatory disorder due to scratching, and characterized by circumscribed areas of thickened and very itchy skin.

CAUSE

This is unknown.

Psychological factors usually play a part. The condition might be explained as an extension of the scratching of the head or face which often occurs at the end of a day's work when owing to fatigue problems appear to be bigger than they are. Mild nervous tension may be sufficient to trigger off the desire to scratch and produce the disease. Other nervous features commonly exist, such as nail or lip-biting, or chain-smoking of cigarettes.

PATHOLOGY

A thickening of all layers of the epidermis may be seen, a little oedema, and a dermal lymphocytic infiltrate.

CLINICAL FEATURES

Itching is intermittent and sometimes very severe.

The onset is insidious, itching and scratching preceding the appearance of any lesions. Papules are first seen, which become confluent to form circumscribed patches of varying shapes and sizes. The colour is red or reddish brown and the surface may be covered with an uneven layer of superficial scales (Plate 16).

The sites commonly affected are the nape of the neck (especially in women), the outer sides of the forearms, the calves of the legs and the outer side of the ankles; in fact, any area which is easy to scratch. Pruritus of the ano-genital area may also be a symptom of localized neurodermatitis.

Glycosuria is occasionally found, and urine examination should not be omitted.

DIAGNOSIS

The disease must be distinguished from *lichen planus*, the lesions of which are purplish, distinctly shiny, and more discrete.

Contact dermatitis, in which the duration and onset are swifter, can be excluded by taking a careful history.

TREATMENT

If the patient can be made to stop scratching, the lesion will heal and this must be made clear to the patient. In investigating a possible psychological cause, it is important to realize that it may have arisen from an episode in the past, such as nursing a dying parent for a long time, sailing through stormy matrimonial seas, or attempts to dodge the tax-man, and the relationship of cause and effect is more real than apparent. In many instances the cause is co-existent and must be treated.

Tranquillizers during the day, and hypnotics at night may be required to prevent the undoing of the improvement which local measures have produced. These may be in the form of intralesional injections of hydrocortisone on several occasions, or the application when practical (i.e. on the arms or legs) of a steroid cream under an occlusive dressing. Superficial X-rays are also useful in selected cases.

PROGNOSIS
Recurrences are common, no matter how successful the therapy appears to have been.

Dermatitis Artefacta

This term describes self-inflicted lesions induced by hysteria or a neurosis which vary in type from a redness to ulceration. The notable feature about the condition is the absence of complete resemblance to any order disorder, and the curious shapes of the lesions.

CAUSES
Hysteria
This comprises the main group. The patient may deny knowing how the lesions developed, and he may, in fact, not know their cause.

Psychoses
Schizophrenics and paranoiacs may mutilate themselves without any obvious motive.

Malingerers
These patients produce the lesions with a motive such as avoiding work which they dislike.

Agents
These may be such substances as carbolic acid, alkalis, cigarettes, matches or sandpaper. They are ingeniously hidden, and it often requires hospitalization before the cause and diagnosis are definitely discovered.

CLINICAL FEATURES
The lesions have an artificial and curiously bizarre appearance possessing angles and edges not associated with the lesions of any other disorder (Fig. 26). Their severity depends on the agent used; severe burns, deep scars, and ragged ulcers may be seen.

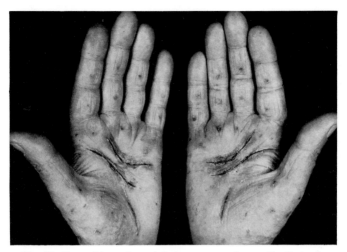

FIG. 26. Dermatitis artefacta, injurious agent unknown (Institute of Dermatology, University of London).

TREATMENT

This is usually difficult and depends on the type of patient, if hysterical, admission to hospital is often necessary. The patient should be carefully watched and the lesions enclosed in occlusive bandages. Lesions developing later on another limb tend to confirm the presumptive diagnosis. The patient should be kept from suspecting the purpose for admission to hospital until proof is definite. Even when the patient is aware of the doctor's diagnosis, lesions may continue to be produced.

For psychotic patients, psychotherapy is required. For malingerers merely to catch the patient producing the lesion is enough to end the disorder.

Trichotillomania

This disorder is characterized by an uncontrollable desire to pull out one's own hair.

CAUSE

Emotional factors are always present. Mild or severe frustrations and anxieties may exist, or more rarely, a true psychosis may be present.

The disease usually affects children but is not unknown in adults.

CLINICAL FEATURES

Usually in one area of the scalp there is a patch of relative baldness with broken off but otherwise normal hairs.

DIAGNOSIS

This disorder must be distinguished from *alopecia areata* and *ringworm*.

In the first case, exclamation-mark hairs will be found (see p. 226) and in the second case, the fungus.

TREATMENT

Children usually grow out of the habit without any special treatment, but adults may require psychotherapy.

Neurotic Excoriations

A disorder in which scars are produced by the patient picking at the skin.

CAUSE

Emotional factors are always present and more often than not are features of hysteria. Women are more prone to the condition than men, and 20–30 is the commonest age group.

CLINICAL FEATURES

Lesions occur on any site accessible to the fingers.

TREATMENT

Suggestion or psychotherapy are usually partially or wholly effective.

CHAPTER 9

Bacterial Diseases

Impetigo: Boil: Folliculitis barbae:
Syphilis: Congenital Syphilis: Tuberculosis:
Lupus vulgaris: Papulo-Necrotic Tuberculid:
Erythema induratum: Tuberculosis verrucosa: Erythrasma:
Anthrax: Leprosy

Introduction

Bacterial infections of the skin are recognized clinically by the presence of crusted lesions, consisting of dried exudate. The infection may be the primary cause of the skin disease, or it may be superimposed on another skin disease.

Coagulase positive staphylococci are the commonest cause of bacterial infections of the skin. The staphylococcus aureus is present in the nostrils of nearly 50 per cent of the population and in the body creases of at least 10 per cent. These areas are therefore a common source of infection.

Other well-known organisms are capable of producing bacterial skin infections; these may be streptococci, coliform bacilli, pseudomonas and proteus, and more rarely, the Klebs–Loeffler bacillus.

The treatment of bacterial infections has of course been revolutionized by the use of antibiotics. The treatment of skin diseases differs from other diseases in that sulphonamide, penicillin, neomycin or chloramphenicol creams or ointments must *not* be prescribed as these antibiotics, when used locally, are liable to initiate a sensitizing dermatitis which will be far more troublesome to deal with than the original disease. Other antibiotics such as the tetra- or oxytetracyclines are just as effective and simple to use in topical form.

Impetigo

This is a contagious, superficially inflammatory disease, characterized by thin-walled vesicles and bullae, which rupture and form honey-coloured crusts (Fig. 27). They are caused predominantly by

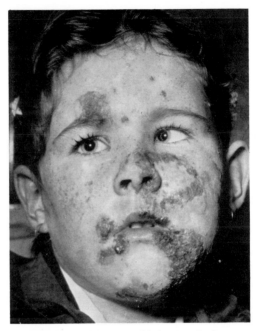

FIG. 27. Impetigo contagiosa. Crusted lesions on the face, secondary to a septic focus in the nose.

Staphylococcus aureus in the U.K., and by β haemolytic streptococci in the U.S.A. The disease is less contagious in adults than in the children who are more commonly troubled by it.

PREDISPOSING CAUSES
These are infected nostrils or ears, dirty finger-nails or towels, or infection from an existing condition such as pediculosis capitis, scabies or eczematous conditions.

PATHOLOGY

The vesicle or bulla arises just below the horny layer and contains polymorphs, lymphocytes and fibrin.

CLINICAL FEATURES

Itching is quite common and the resulting scratching leads to inoculation of the disease elsewhere.

The size of the lesion varies from a pea to a coin. The shape of the lesion is roughly circular, but gyrate lesions also occur. Sites most commonly affected are the face and ears.

COURSE

Untreated the disease tends to clear up spontaneously in a month or so.

DIAGNOSIS

When lesions are circinate, ringworm may be considered, but here the lesions are never so crusted or red and fungi are found in scrapings.

TREATMENT

When the diagnosis is made, great care should be taken to prevent other members of the household using the patient's towels, napkins, etc.

An antibiotic ointment, to which the organisms have proved to be sensitive, applied twice daily will clear the disease within a week. Possible sources of infection, such as the nose and ears, should be examined and treated similarly when necessary. When the condition is extensive, systemic antibiotics should be given to avoid the possibility of acute glomerulo-nephritis.

Boil

Furuncle

A boil is an acute painful infection of a hair follicle caused by staphylococcus pyogenes. A *carbuncle* is a conglomerated mass of boils.

PREDISPOSING CAUSES

These are eczema, scabies, pediculosis, and seborrhoea which, being itchy conditions, result in the inoculation of staphylococci by scratching. Diabetes mellitus, alcoholism, anaemia and lowered states of health from, for example, overwork, also predispose to boils.

Latent foci in the nose, ears, under the nails or on the perineum should be considered.

Adolescent boys are more affected than girls.

CLINICAL FEATURES

The onset is quite sudden. The skin becomes red round a follicle; tenderness, heat and oedema follow, and the centre becomes yellow with pus. It soon discharges and the yellowish-green core usually follows. Scars are a common remainder. Sites commonly affected are the back of the neck, the axillae, the buttocks and the thighs.

TREATMENT

Penicillin may be employed in doses of 250 mg four times a day in tablet form, for 4 or 5 days. Should this fail, as it occasionally does, a broad spectrum antibiotic such as a tetracycline (Aureomycin) or an oxytetracycline (Terramycin) should be used in the same dosage. Local applications are not useful, but the painful boil should be protected from trauma by a dressing.

Prognosis

A tendency for boils to recur, on and off, for some months, is not uncommon, in those subject to them. The antibiotic ointments to which the bacteria are sensitive should be applied to the areas where latent foci are apt to be found (*vide supra*), daily for 2–3 weeks. Hexachlorophene (pHisoHex) in a daily bath, and dusting with chlorhexidine (Hibitane) powder afterwards are useful in forming an anti-bacterial barrier, although contra-indicated in the care of children.

Folliculitis barbae

Sycosis barbae

This is a chronic staphylococcal infection of the hair follicles of the beard and moustache areas. It is also known as barber's rash.

Although the title emphasizes involvement of the beard, other hairy areas such as the thighs may also become affected. On the face, the condition is usually secondary to a nasal infection.

CLINICAL FEATURES
The onset is insidious. The lesions are follicular, each pustule being pierced by a hair and once established, the spread to other follicles is rapid. Blepharitis is a common accompaniment.

TREATMENT
This apparently straightfoward condition is often difficult to treat, but is best approached by the eradication of focal sepsis, such as bad teeth or infected tonsils. Prophylactic measures regarding other members of the household (see impetigo) must be taken.

External
Apply the antibiotic to which the organisms are sensitive, e.g. tetracycline (Aureomycin) or oxytetracycline (Terramycin) ointment twice daily for at least a month.

Internal
The same drugs are used, e.g. Aureomycin or Terramycin 250 mg t.d.s. for 1 week, and then b.d.s. for 1 week.

PROGNOSIS
The avoidance of recurrences, which are apt to occur, depends on meticulous cleanliness of shaving and other toilet equipment, such as towels, and the daily application of hexachlorophene (pHisoHex) lotion, after shaving.

Syphilis

Lues

This is an infectious and contagious disease, caused by *Treponema pallidum* (*Spirochaeta pallida*), which is capable of invading every organ of the body and producing such protean manifestations that it is likely to imitate many other diseases in many ways. W.H.O. however reported increases again in 70 of 105 countries who reported in 1965.

Since the introduction of antibiotics there has been a great reduction in the number of cases all over the world, and this being so, diagnosis of syphilis of the skin often depends on consciously remembering its existence.

The synonym lues, and its adjective luetic, are useful words to use in front of patients when discussing the possibility of a diagnosis of syphilis, and the patient should not be informed until the diagnosis is an absolute certainty, for the consequences to the patient are very great.

CAUSE

The organism *Treponema pallidum* is a delicate threadlike spiral parasite, 6–15 μ in length and with pointed ends. The number of spirals varies between 8 and 24. It can bend on itself without losing its spiral shape, open and close like a concertina, and act like a screw in its movements.

Transmission

In acquired syphilis this may be by direct infection through sexual intercourse (95 per cent of cases), less commonly by kissing, and rarely through contaminated drinking vessels, or the communal use of such things as tattooing needles, or wind instruments.

Congenital syphilis is transmitted by an infected mother, usually in the early stages of the disease, by transplacental passage of the organism into the blood stream of the foetus. This takes place most commonly after the sixth month of pregnancy. The father cannot transmit congenital syphilis.

PATHOLOGY

The essential lesion in all phases of syphilis is the same, being strikingly characterized by peri-vascular round cell infiltration, mainly lymphocytic, and to a lesser extent by plasma, and mononuclear cells. Granulomatous and giant-cell formation occurs in later stages, and all these changes give rise to the sensation of induration derived from palpating (with a protected finger) a syphilitic lesion.

The primary chancre and the lesions of secondary syphilis contain many spirochaetes, but in the tertiary or gummatous lesions the spirochaetes are sparse.

CLINICAL FEATURES

There are 3 stages which are quite distinct in the time they occur and the features they present.

Primary stage occurs between 10 and 28 days after infection (the limits are 9–90 days). The primary lesion or chancre is an indurated, inflammatory, papular lesion, usually ulcerated and covered with scanty exudate. The site most commonly affected is the coronal sulcus, but any area of the penis may be involved, including the interior of the urethra, and the ano-rectal area in homosexuals. In women, the labium majora or minora are the commonest areas, but no area is immune including the cervix. In a small percentage of cases, the lips or other facial areas may be the site of a chancre. The site of the genital chancre in women often results in it being overlooked, so that secondary syphilis is the first intimation they have of the disease.

Regional adenitis is common, and malaise is often present.

COURSE

Untreated, a chancre will resolve, and the secondary stage will be the first sign of the disease. Approximately 25 per cent of patients give no history of a primary lesion.

INVESTIGATIONS

Treponema pallidum is found by microscopical dark-ground examination of exudate from a lesion, or from fluid aspirated from an enlarged regional lymph node.

The Wassermann reaction (W.R.) is usually positive 4–6 weeks after infection, and invariably during the second stage. Technical errors may occur and positive results should always be confirmed by repetition. It should be noted that the W.R. is often positive in other conditions, e.g. yaws, leprosy, glandular fever and malaria, and does not therefore invariably indicate syphilis.

DIAGNOSIS

This is made by the investigations described, and the clinical signs.

Scabies of the penis is associated with itching and burrows may be found. *Herpes genitalis* is a very superficial lesion. *Chancroid* lesions are painful and not indurated, and uncommon in this country. An *epithelioma* has a rolled edge, and its evolution is extremely slow.

A chancre of the nipple must be differentiated from *Paget's disease* of the nipple, a digital one from *paronychia*, while *haemorrhoids* or *fissures* may closely mimic an anal chancre.

SECONDARY STAGE

This occurs between 6 weeks and 2 years after the appearance of the chancre, and lasts about 2 years. About 75 per cent of patients show skin lesions, 50 per cent have generalized lymphadenopathy, a third have oral and tonsillar lesions, and a very small number have involvement of the nervous system, bones, eyes or abdominal viscera.

CLINICAL FEATURES

These are usually vague, and include headaches, nausea, vomiting anorexia, bone, muscle and joint pains, laryngitis, tonsillitis and fever, usually 100°–101°F (38°–39°C). Symptoms precede the skin lesions, which are called syphilids.

The skin lesions vary in appearance and character, imitating many diseases, although they are never vesicular or bullous in acquired syphilis. (In early congenital syphilis, they may be.) The lesions do not itch, with the rare exception of some papular lesions in coloured patients.

Lesions first to appear are macular, or maculo-papular, and are the commonest seen.

Early Lesions	*Late Lesions*	
Macular	Annular	
Maculo-papular	Pustular	All uncommon
Papular	Psoriasiform	

Macular lesions (Fig. 28)
These vary in size from 0·5 to 2 cm, and are round. Their colour is rose or red and may only be seen in natural light and at a distance. Sites commonly affected are the shoulders, chest, back and arms. They may persist for only a few days, or change into papular lesions.

Papular lesions
These develop from macules, or appear spontaneously as the first

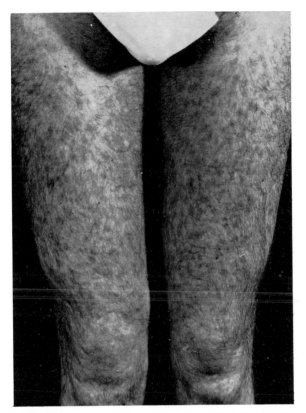

Fig. 28. Secondary syphilid: macular lesions (Institute of Dermatology, University of London).

sign of the secondary stage. Similar in shape and size to macular lesions, the colour is coppery. Sites commonly affected are trunk, arms and legs, palms (Plate 17), soles and face. On the hair-line of the forehead and temples, papules may congregate like a garland, which has been called caustically the corona veneris. They may be scaly and, above all, are definitely indurated when palpated.

Moist papular lesions also occur, better known as *condylomata lata*. They are shiny, fleshy, flat, firm or soft, poorly or well-defined lesions. The sites affected are the ano-genital, axillary and sub-mammary areas, between the fingers and toes, and at the angles of the mouth.

Moist papular lesions on the mucous membranes of the oral cavity, tongue, palate and pharynx, are known as *mucous patches*. They are about half an inch across and are irregular in shape; in the pharynx they are long, narrow and eroded and called *snail track ulcers*. The surface of the lesions is covered with a greyish film, which can be scraped off, leaving a pink area which does not bleed. These moist papular lesions are crawling with spirochaetes.

Other signs are

1. Alopecia, which is not common, but when it does occur is patchy, involving the scalp, beard and eyebrows.
2. Jaundice may occur in severe infections.
3. Secondary anaemia, and a leucocytosis of 10,000–20,000 per ml with 50–80 per cent lymphocytes.
4. Generalized lymphadenopathy.
5. Atrophy of the skin where lesions have healed may occur.

DIAGNOSIS

This is made by finding the *Treponema pallidum* from the skin or mucous membrane lesions, and a positive W.R.

Macular syphilis must be differentiated from the acute *exanthemata* such as *measles*, *drug eruptions*, *pityriasis rosea* and *glandular fever*; *papular syphilis* from *psoriasis*, *seborrhoeic dermatitis*, *urticaria*, *lichen planus*, and *drug eruptions*; *pustular syphilis* from other pustular conditions, including *bromide* and *iodide eruptions*; *mucous patches* from *Vincent's angina*, *tonsillitis*, *aphthous ulcers*, and *lichen planus*.

TERTIARY STAGE

This occurs 2–30 years after infection. Patients can often give no history of a primary or secondary stage. *T. pallida* are present, but in very small numbers, and can often only be demonstrated by animal inoculation. Lesions are all gummatous. There are three types of gummata: (1) nodular, (2) squamous, (3) single.

CLINICAL FEATURES

Nodular lesions vary in size from a pin-head to a pea. They are reddish and well defined. Distribution is asymmetrical. Squamous gummatous lesions may be large, spreading across the body. Their shape is variable, being polycyclic or arciform and well defined, with activity apparent on the edge.

Single lesions start as smooth painless swellings which break down to form ulcers, which look as if they had been produced by a metal punch. In time they may involve underlying tissues. These particularly attack the leg, scalp, face, and sterno-clavicular areas, They may also attack the mucous membranes of the mouth, throat, and nose, being diffuse or localized.

Other signs are
1. Bursitis of elbow joint, acromial process of the scapula, and extensor tendons of the fingers.
2. Cardiovascular, C.N.S., and visceral complications.

DIAGNOSIS

This is made by the history, and serological tests. Standard tests for syphilis such as the V.D.R.L. tests are not specific, as they detect the presence of a substance called 'reagin', which can be present in other diseases. They are negative in the incubation period, but are nearly always positive 10–14 days after the appearance of the primary chancre. The W.R. may also be done, but is gradually becoming out-dated.

Tests based on treponemal antigens are much more specific. The first of these tests to be introduced, the Treponemal Immobilization Test or T.P.I., is the most accurate, but is technically difficult to perform and hence expensive. The Fluorescent Treponemal Antibody Test (F.T.A.), which makes use of dead treponemes, is, however, very specific and technically much simpler to perform. It is also inexpensive.

These treponemal tests should not be used routinely. Their main use is to confirm the diagnosis of syphilis when the standard tests for syphilis are positive in the absence of signs or history of the disease.

Tertiary syphilis must be differentiated from *lupus vulgaris*, from *leprosy*, and *carcinomata*.

TREATMENT

Prophylactic

1. Education of the public, which at present is inadequate.
2. Condoms, in 'at risk' situations, though they may not afford complete protection.

Curative

All early cases of syphilis respond rapidly to 600,000 units of procaine penicillin G. given intramuscularly daily for 10 days. The same treatment is effective for all forms of late syphilis, except neurosyphilis, when the treatment should be continued for 3 weeks.

In penicillin-sensitive patients tetracycline hydrochloride 500 mg 6-hourly for 10–14 days is probably the most effective drug. It should not be given during pregnancy, and in these circumstances erythromycin is probably the best alternative.

Congenital Syphilis

As already stated, infection is contracted from the child's mother. Paternal transmission from the semen does not occur.

Prematurity and neonatal death are common. The signs of congenital syphilis usually occur within a month of birth, but in rare cases, are delayed for 15–20 years.

New cases of congenital syphilis are rarely seen now because of routine ante-natal W.R. tests in this country.

CLINICAL FEATURES

In the early stages, these are coryza, nasal discharge, snuffles, wasting and insomnia.

Lesions may be macular, papular or bullous. When bullae break, ulcers form. Any site may be affected, but the buttocks, the palms and soles are invariably attacked. The bullae contain spirochetes.

Linear fissures may occur at the angles of the mouth and healing of them in later life appears as rhagades. Peri-anal condylomata appear a little later; infants in this phase are extremely contagious.

Other signs are the saddle-nose, saucer-shaped facies, sometimes painful and not always symmetrical hydrarthrosis (Clutton's joints), Hutchinson's triad of interstitial keratitis, deafness and notched incisors of the second dentition, besides other signs reflecting involvement of other organs.

TREATMENT

Curative
600,000 units of penicillin for 10 days, and if there is evidence of neurosyphilis, a 3-week course is necessary.

Chronic Gonococcal Dermatitis

This condition tends to occur most frequently in those patients in whom gonorrhoea is initially latent, and is seen particularly in women with genital or pharyngeal gonorrhoea, or homosexual men with rectal or pharyngeal infections. The illness usually presents with a low fever, malaise and arthralgia or actual arthritis, particularly of the joints of the lower limb. A typical feature is the development of haemorrhagic vesicles or pustules which develop around infected joints. Many such patients are treated with antibiotics in general practice without a diagnosis being made. If treatment is not given the septicaemic process may progress to a 'septic' stage with multiple joint involvement, rigors and even hepatic involvement.

DIAGNOSIS

This is made by isolating the gonococcus from material taken from urethra, cervix, rectum and/or oropharynx, rather than attempting to culture the organism from the blood, though this can frequently be done.

TREATMENT

Intra-muscular penicillin for a week or ten days is usually all that is required. Co-trimoxazole by mouth is equally effective in the rare infection which is resistant to penicillin, or when the patient gives a history of hyper-sensitivity to the drug.

Tuberculosis

Tuberculosis, once the scourge of humanity and the tragic source of pathos in novel and opera, has declined sensationally, at any rate in the Western Hemisphere. The improvement has been partly due to the introduction of effective chemotherapy.

Tuberculosis of the skin is now a rare disease in developed countries. It exists in two principal forms:

I. *Localized*
    (a) Lupus vulgaris
    (b) Chancre
    (c) Tuberculosis verrucosa   } Rare
    (d) Tuberculous gumma

II. *Haematogenous forms, known as tuberculids*
    (a) Papulo-necrotic
    (b) Erythema induratum
    (c) Lichenoid   } Rare
    (d) Acne agminata

Lupus Vulgaris

In this type, the tubercle bacillus is directly inoculated into the skin, or reaches it either by spreading from underlying infected glands or joints, or via the lymphatics from an upper respiratory infection. It is commoner in women than men.

PATHOLOGY

The tubercles typical of tuberculosis with epithelioid and Langhans cells, lymphocytes, plasma cells and caseation can be seen in the dermis. In the healing stage, extensive fibrosis is apparent.

CLINICAL FEATURES

The onset is insidious. The first lesion is a deep nodule, slowly forming a plaque as it coalesces with neighbouring lesions. The lesion may ultimately ulcerate, or atrophy, or hypertrophy. The shape of the lesion is always irregular, and the surface may be covered with an adherent crust. The colour is yellowish red, but when a watch-glass is pressed on it (this examination is called diascopy) the lesion becomes white, and the nodules appear as brown apple-jelly-like spots in the centre. The sites commonly attacked are the nose, cheeks and ears. In pre-chemotherapeutic days, the nose was destroyed. Large lesions can also be found on the trunk, hands and feet, in some cases. The buccal mucous membrane lesions appear as grey granulomatous patches; the tongue when attacked has large painful fissures.

Complications
Carcinoma *in situ* occurs in 1 or 2 per cent of cases.

DIAGNOSIS
This is made by the indolence of the lesion, the 'apple-jelly nodules', the tuberculin patch test and biopsy. The disease must be distinguished from *syphilis*, in which lesions are progressive, from *lupus erythematosus* whose lesions are covered by tiny horny plugged scales, *psoriasis* which shows heaped-up scales and involvement of the extensors, and *sarcoidosis* in which lesions evolve far more rapidly and are multiple.

TREATMENT
Isoniazid (Iso-nicotinic acid hydrazide) is the drug of choice. The average adult dose is 300–400 mg daily for 6 months, and then for 3 months after cessation of all activity. Toxic effects are rare, and can be minimized by giving pyridoxine 100 mg daily.

Isoniazide is usually combined with streptomycin or ethambutol. In obstinate cases, it may be combined with rifampicin. The latter drug stains the urine red. Purpuric and pemphigus-like eruptions have been reported following its use.

Papulo-Necrotic Tuberculid

Tuberculid means a tuberculous condition in which the presence of tubercle bacilli cannot be demonstrated, although the pathology of the lesion resembles tuberculosis. This type of tuberculid, as the words imply, means a condition presenting a papule with (central) necrosis.

They are found in young people and appear in crops as small round discrete lesions on the extensor surfaces of the arms and legs. On healing, scars will be found.

TREATMENT
The same as for lupus vulgaris.

Erythema Induratum

Bazin's Disease

This condition is characterized by symmetrical red indurated nodules on the backs of the legs, and occasionally elsewhere. It predominates in females, between the ages of 10 and 20.

PATHOLOGY

This shows a non-specific or tuberculoid infiltrate in the lower part of the dermis. Proliferative changes occur, and caseation which accounts for the clinical breakdown of the lesions.

CLINICAL FEATURES

The lesions are notably painless.

The nodules break down, ulcerate and leave scars. The edges of the ulcers are steep or undermined. The lesions may persist for months.

DIAGNOSIS

The indolence, symmetry and painlessness of the lesions distinguish this disease from *erythema nodosum* which is a painful condition, without ulceration, *nodular syphilid* which will reveal other signs of the disease, and *chilblains* which are tender, and rarely ulcerate.

Treat as for lupus vulgaris.

Tuberculosis Verrucosa

This is a warty condition resulting from accidental inoculation whilst handling infected materials from autopsies, or meat. It is also known as a prosector's wart.

Erythrasma

This mildly inflammatory condition is caused by a diphtheroid, *C. minutissimum*, which is gram-positive, as well as other species, e.g. of the Bacillus or Streptomyces variety.

CLINICAL FEATURES

Slightly inflamed, dry, slightly scaly, well-defined, macular lesions develop in the genito-crural area; and also in the axillary, infra-mammary, or interdigital areas of the feet.

DIAGNOSIS

Affected areas show a coral red fluorescence under Wood's light, due to the production of a porphyrin. Its clinical similarity to tinea cruris may be very misleading (page 139).

TREATMENT

Erythromycin or oxytetracyclines by mouth can be effective. Alternatively, 2 per cent sodium fusidate ointment, or clotrimazole cream (Canesten) or miconazole cream (Dermonistat) may be applied twice daily for 2 weeks.

Anthrax

This rare condition is also known as a malignant pustule, but is only occasionally fatal. It is an acute infection caused by the anthrax bacillus, and characterized by a gangrenous carbuncular lesion, accompanied by constitutional symptoms.

It is common in the Middle and Far East, and very rare in Europe.

PREDISPOSING CAUSES

As anthrax is a disease of animals, cattle-men, woolsorters, tanners and butchers carry the occupational risk of contracting it.

The disease may also be contracted through the hair of shaving brushes. It is common in the Middle and Far East but rare in Europe.

PATHOLOGY

The epidermis is destroyed and replaced by an ulcer on which bacilli can be found in large numbers.

CLINICAL FEATURES

Incubation period is 12–72 hours. Headache and high fever are followed, if untreated, by prostration and delirium. A small red papule, about the size of a flea-bite, becomes progressively vesicular, pustular and bullous, and then breaks down.

DIAGNOSIS

This is made by isolating *B. anthracis*, and thus distinguishing the condition from a *carbuncle*, or a *chancre*.

TREATMENT

Penicillin or oxytetracyclines are effective orally.

PROGNOSIS

This is good when an early diagnosis has been made, otherwise poor.

Leprosy

Hansen's Disease or Infection; Hanseniasis

A chronic mycobacterial disease, infectious in some cases, primarily affecting peripheral nerves and secondarily affecting skin and certain other tissues.

CAUSE

Mycobacterium leprae is the generally accepted cause of leprosy but this is unproven as all attempts to infect volunteers have failed. The bacterium, discovered by Hansen in Norway in 1873, is similar in appearance to *M. tuberculosis* but the fact that it is less acid-fast and alcohol-fast must be taken into account when Ziehl-Neelsen method of staining is being employed. Mode of transmission is now believed to be by droplets from the upper respiratory tracts of persons suffering from the lepromatous form of the disease (see below) prior to treatment; hence leprosy is often seen in families even though congenital transmission does not occur. It is doubtful if the older hypothesis of skin to skin contact can be sustained. Incubation period is between 2 and 7 years.

PATHOLOGY

Changes in the tissues vary according to the resistance of the infected individual. Tuberculoid leprosy is seen in those with good resistance (cell-mediated immunity), and a tuberculoid histology is found in an affected nerve or in a skin lesion, but acid-fast bacilli (A.F.B.) are absent; tuberculoid granulomata have been described in liver and lymph glands in some cases, but have not caused symptoms.

Lepromatous leprosy is seen in those with poor resistance, and histological changes consist of histiocytes and macrophages (the latter are histiocytes containing leprosy bacilli). Scanty round cells (lymphocytes) and plasma cells may be seen, but epithelioid and giant cells are absent. Macrophages containing a predominance of dead bacilli appear as foamy cells in H. & E. sections because of fatty content, and staining by special methods such as Fite-Faraco is necessary to demonstrate leprosy bacilli. These are seen in large numbers, lying singly or in clumps of various sizes. Spherical masses of bacilli are commonly seen, and are macrophages packed with bacilli; these are known as globi. These changes can be seen in many tissues in addition to nerves and skin, such as skeletal muscle, mucosa of upper respiratory tract, reticuloendothelial system, eyes and testes.

Borderline (dimorphous) leprosy occurs in those who, immunologically speaking, are between the two 'polar' types just described, hence the dissemination of the infection in the body, the histological changes, and the numbers of bacilli in the affected tissues, depend on the position of the patient in the borderline spectrum (Fig. 29).

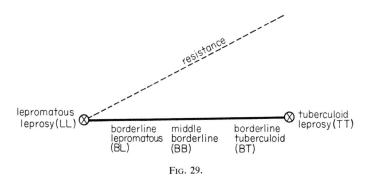

FIG. 29.

Indeterminate leprosy is an uncommon and transient form of the disease which may be self-limiting or may evolve into one of the determinate types described above. Histological appearances in the skin are slight and non-specific.

CLINICAL FEATURES

Skin lesions in leprosy avoid the warmer parts of the skin such as the hairy scalp, axillae, groins and perineum, and favour the cooler parts such as face and ears, arms, backs of hands and fingers, buttocks and legs.

The typical lesion in tuberculoid leprosy is a plaque which is erythematous, usually single, with raised and well defined edges from which there is a gradual slope towards a flattened and hypo-pigmented centre (Plate 18). The surface is dry, hairless, insensitive, sometimes scaly, and a thickened peripheral nerve is usually palpable in the vicinity. In fact, damage to a peripheral nerve, causing sensory or motor disturbance (or both), may precede the skin lesion. Less commonly the lesion is a macule (level with the skin), erythematous in light skins and hypopigmented (never *de*pigmented) in dark skins, with sometimes a coppery tint. The macule is well defined and has a dry, hairless and insensitive surface. In rare cases there may be a purely neural form with sensory loss and/or motor disturbance, and thickening of the affected nerve is diagnostic.

Lesions of lepromatous leprosy are small, multiple, faintly erythematous, shiny, scattered bilaterally and symmetrically, and show no impairment of sensation or hair growth (Plate 19). These are likely to be of different types, all of which can be seen in the same patient—macules, plaques, papules and nodules. Nerves are not thickened in the earlier stages (unless there has been a down-grading from a previous borderline form) but become fibrotic and thickened after many years of treatment. Other features which develop as the *untreated* disease advances are oedema of legs and feet, nasal blockage and bleeding, hoarse voice, leprous keratitis and iridocyclitis, thinning or loss of eyebrows and eyelashes, thickening of ear lobes and of skin of face with deepening of the lines in the forehead (leonine facies), loosening or loss of upper incisor teeth, 'glove and stocking' anaesthesia, shortening of fingers and trophic ulceration of feet due to repeated painless trauma, and, in males, testicular atrophy. It should be noted that oedema of legs and/or nasal symptoms may be the first manifestations of lepromatous leprosy. This is the only type of leprosy which may shorten life expectancy, the cause being renal damage in the form of chronic glomerulonephritis, chronic interstitial nephritis, or renal amyloido-sis. At one time it was thought that pulmonary tuberculosis was a common cause of death, but this was a false impression conveyed by the high incidence of tuberculosis in leprosaria; recent observations on leprosy out-patients have shown that the incidence of tuberculosis is no higher than in the general population.

Lesions of borderline leprosy are intermediate in number and in clinical features between the 'polar' types, and often take the form of annular lesions (Plate 20) or of raised erythematous bands forming bizarre shapes. Plaques have outer edges which are ill defined in parts, and some have 'punched-out' centres which are characteristic (Plate 21). Well-defined hypopigmented macules may be present in dark-skinned patients. Lesions show a variable amount of anaesthesia, and thickening of peripheral nerves is usually present from the very beginning. In fact, there may be a prolonged pure polyneuritic phase before the appearance of skin lesions. On the tuberculoid side of the spectrum lesions are fewer and drier, have more hair loss, are more insensitive, have fewer bacilli in smears and biopsies, and vice versa. Damage to structures other than skin and nerves will not be manifest even though bacilli may be present in lymph glands, liver, or in striated muscle.

The patient with indeterminate leprosy, usually a child, presents with a single macule, erythematous in light skins and hypopigmented in dark skins, and sensory impairment is slight or absent. It is here that the histamine test can be of real value in diagnosis by showing a weak or absent flare.

REACTIONAL STATES IN LEPROSY

There are two distinct types of reactional state (reaction or lepra reaction), and precipitating factors include anti-leprosy drugs, intercurrent infection, various types of vaccination, severe physical or mental stress, injury, surgical operation, pregnancy and parturition. One type of reaction, which we can call Type 1 lepra reaction, principally seen in borderline leprosy, is characterized by swelling and redness of skin lesions and by pain and swelling in one or more nerves; oedema of the extremities is common but fever and constitutional disturbance are unusual. Sometimes new lesions rapidly appear. This type of reaction is due to an extremely rapid change in cell-mediated immunity, and is called upgrading or reversal when immunity increases and downgrading when it decreases. An upgrading reaction is likely to occur during the first 6 months of treatment, especially if dosage of anti-leprosy drug is increased too rapidly, and although it signifies a rapid move towards cure it may have disastrous consequences in the form of crippling nerve damage such as facial paralysis, claw hand, or dropped foot. The other type of reaction, known as Type 2 lepra reaction or ENL reaction, is confined to lepromatous leprosy and is a form of antigen–antibody reaction known as an immune complex syndrome, the antigen being the protein liberated when leprosy bacilli are killed, and the antibody being present in tissues (especially in small blood vessels) and in the circulation. This type of reaction, unlike Type 1 lepra reaction, usually occurs after the first 6 months of treatment and when the majority of leprosy bacilli are dead, i.e. when they are seen as fragmented and granular bacilli in skin smears and biopsies. One of the classical features is *erythema nodosum leprosum* (ENL) consisting of transient erythematous nodules and patches occurring in crops on any part of the skin but particularly on face, arms and thighs, usually fading in a few days and being replaced by fresh lesions, and sometimes becoming bullous or necrotic. Other manifestations include fever, oedema of extremities, neuritis, myositis, swollen joints, painful and tender tibiae, tenderness and swelling of one or more lymph glands, epistaxis, iridocyclitis, epididymo-orchitis, and proteinuria. In both types of reaction swelling of nerves may be associated with signs of nerve damage such as sensory loss and/or muscle paralysis. Pain in affected nerves is greater by night than by day and is the biggest problem in management.

INVESTIGATIONS

Two tests of paramount importance in diagnosing leprosy lesions are:

   (1) testing for sensation with a pin, a wisp of cotton wool, and with hot and cold test tubes; and

   (2) making smears which will be stained for A.F.B.

With these two tests nearly all leprosy lesions can be diagnosed, for tuberculoid and borderline-tuberculoid lesions are anaesthetic and devoid of bacilli, mid-borderline and borderline-lepromatous lesions combine impaired sensation with the presence of bacilli, and lepromatous lesions are rich in bacilli. Nasal scrapings are of value in deciding if a lepromatous patient is potentially infectious, but are of little value in diagnosis as they are negative in the tuberculoid and borderline types; nor are they of value in follow-up testing as bacilli disappear from the nasal mucosa long before they disappear from the skin.

To make a *skin smear*, the lesion is cleaned with ether and a fold is gripped between thumb and forefinger of the left hand to render it avascular. With a small-bladed scalpel (size 15 Bard Parker blade) an incision is made 5 mm long and 3 mm deep; the blade is then turned at right angles to the cut, and, without relaxing finger pressure, the wound is scraped several times in one direction. Fluid and pulp from the dermis collects on one side of the blade and is gently smeared on to a glass slide. A *skin biopsy* will help in confirming the diagnosis and in classification.

Histamine test: A drop of 1 in 1000 histamine diphosphate solution is placed in the centre of the hypopigmented macule and a pin-prick is made through the drop. The bright flare which appears after 1–2 minutes in normal skin will be depressed or absent in a leprosy macule because of damage to autonomic nerves in the skin.

A *lepromin test* is a non-specific test which is valueless in diagnosis but is of value in classifying a case of leprosy, the reaction being strongly positive in the tuberculoid type, negative in the lepromatous type, and intermediate in borderline. The test is unpredictable in indeterminate leprosy.

Blood changes in leprosy are confined to the lepromatous type, and the commonest findings are anaemia (normocytic and normo-chromic), increase in serum globulin, and a raised E.S.R. Other findings are less common and include false positive Wassermann reactions, and positive tests for thyroglobulin antibodies, L.E. cells, antinuclear factor, rheumatoid factor, and cold precipitable protein.

TREATMENT

Prophylactic

In the past, segregating leprosy patients was the only method of prophylaxis. Nowadays early diagnosis and effective chemotherapy are all-important as the patient with bacilli in his nasal mucosa is thereby rendered non-infectious relatively quickly and long before the disease is arrested. B.C.G. vaccination is a prophylactic weapon, and should be given to all children at risk and to all tuberculin-negative adults who are likely to come in contact with the disease. Children living under the same roof as a leprosy patient can, in addition, be given a prophylactic course of sulphone for at least 3 years. Improved living conditions, particularly in housing, reduce the amount of close contact within families.

Therapeutic

This should be on an out-patient basis whenever possible as admission to a leprosy hospital has many ill effects on the patient, particularly psychological. Also it hinders control of the disease as many leprosy sufferers will deliberately avoid diagnosis in order not to be removed from their homes and families. Because of the low infectivity of the disease, patients requiring hospital admission for short periods can be admitted to a general hospital ward, and only in the case of a lepromatous patient at the very beginning of treatment need a modified form of barrier nursing be instituted. *Danger to others, if any, arises not from the leprosy patient under treatment but from the undiagnosed case.*

The most widely used anti-leprosy drug, and by far the cheapest, is dapsone (DDS) administered orally. There is no hard and fast dosage scheme, although there is general agreement that 700 mg/week should not be exceeded. The clinician should be very cautious during the first 6 months in tuberculoid and borderline leprosy for fear of precipitating a Type 1 lepra reaction, and dosage should not exceed 25 mg twice a week during this time; thereafter it can be increased to 25 mg daily. Recent research in treating lepromatous leprosy has thrown doubt on Type 2 lepra reaction (ENL) being dosage dependent, and optimum dosage of 50–100 mg daily can be given from the very beginning, especially if bacilli in smears and biopsies are mostly solid-staining (i.e. are living). Another reason for avoiding small doses of dapsone over a long period in treating lepromatous patients (who are notorious for being irregular on treatment) is the risk of encouraging bacterial resistance to the drug, a development which fortunately is not a problem in other types of leprosy. Although dapsone can be given twice a week, or even once a week, the advantage of daily dosage is that out-patients find it easier to remember to take treatment regularly; furthermore, an occasional omission is of little importance. Treatment should be continued for 5 years in tuberculoid leprosy, for 10–15 years in borderline leprosy, and for life in the lepromatous type. Side effects are largely theoretical at this dosage, but include haemolytic anaemia, agranulocytosis, and toxic hepatitis. Other anti-leprosy drugs include certain thiourea compounds such as thiambutosine (Ciba 1906) and thiacetazone (TB1); long-acting sulphonamides; rifampicin; and a riminophenazine derivative known as clofazimine (Lamprene; B 663). The last-named combines an anti-leprosy action as effective as that of dapsone with an anti-inflammatory action which is valuable in controlling Type 2 lepra reaction. Rifampicin should be reserved for the treatment of lepromatous leprosy, and early hopes that it might be capable of eradicating the lepromatous infection have been disappointed; in fact, after a year on rifampicin the patient is no nearer arrest of the disease than is the patient treated with dapsone, and the antibiotic is very expensive. Its real advantage is that it will render a lepromatous patient non-infectious in 2 weeks, and treatment can then be continued with dapsone. Daily dosage for an adult is 600 mg given at least half an hour before breakfast. Immunotherapy is being tried in lepromatous leprosy by injecting lymphocytes or extracts from lymphocytes (transfer factor) derived from patients with tuberculoid leprosy or from healthy donors hypersensitive to lepromin, but is at this stage purely experimental.

TREATMENT OF REACTIONAL STATES

This is one of the most difficult problems in clinical medicine. Those who are inexperienced in managing this condition are advised to reduce dosage of dapsone to 5 mg/day (or 25 mg twice a week) as a first step. Suitable drugs will be required for counteracting anxiety, pain and insomnia, and a short course of trivalent antimony injections can be tried, but corticosteroids will be needed if there is muscle paralysis (threatened or real), epididymo-orchitis, or if there is acute iridocyclitis not responding to local treatment with steroid drops and homatropine. Thalidomide suppresses Type 2 lepra reaction but is obtainable only for therapeutic research; it will never be marketed because of its potential teratogenic effect. Replacing dapsone by clofazimine may facilitate reduction in steroid dosage. Splinting and physiotherapy are required for paralysed muscles.

OTHER TREATMENTS

The care of insensitive hands and feet is important, and regular attention by a chiropodist, together with the supply of suitable footwear, will go far towards preventing plantar ulceration. The lepromatous patient should have regular examination of eyes so that silent iridocyclitis can be diagnosed and treated, while nasal symptoms can be relieved by the regular application of an ointment consisting of Ung. Benovate-N one part and Unguentum Merck two parts. Reconstructive surgery is required for paralysed fingers, foot drop, and hammer toe. Plastic surgery can correct facial disfigurement caused by loss of eyebrows, facial palsy, collapsed nose, ectropion, pendulous ear lobes, and excessive folds of skin. Ichthyotic skin responds to daily application of Calmurid cream after soaking in warm water.

CHAPTER 10

Fungal Diseases

Tinea pedis: T. manuum: T. unguium: T. corporis: T. cruris: T. capitis: Pityriasis versicolor: Candidiasis

Introduction

Fungi are non-photosynthetic entities, and do not contain chlorophyll. They depend on the tissue in which they exist for growth. Many hundreds of fungi abound, yet only a few are capable of producing disease. Those capable of doing so are divided into the superficial and deep species, depending on whether the resulting condition is associated or not with a systemic disease. In this chapter, reference will only be made to the superficial type of fungal infection.

The number of cases of fungal diseases cannot be categorically stated as it varies from one part of the world to another, but in the British Isles it probably accounts for 5 per cent of all cases of skin disease.

Superficial fungi live *on* the skin, and nearly entirely on dead horny tissue, living structures usually being avoided. They digest keratin, the structural basis of the horny layer of the skin, the nails and hair, resulting in disintegration of these structures.

The fungi consist of two parts: (1) the mycelium or vegetative part, made up of filaments or hyphae which acquires food; (2) the spore, or reproductive part, which is a mass of protoplasm surmounted by its wall.

There are three families, or genera, of superficial fungi: Trichophyton, Microsporum, and Epidermophyton. The diseases they cause are neither very infectious nor very contagious, and contraction of the disease depends to a great extent on individual susceptibility and predisposing factors such as hyperidrosis.

Some fungi also cause disease which produces symptoms of

131

cutaneous and/or systemic involvement. Examples of such conditions are actinomycosis, blastomycosis, and histoplasmosis; descriptions of such disorders will be found in larger textbooks.

Tinea

The most important superficial fungi are the ringworm fungi which attack the skin, nails and hair (Fig. 30).

The *diagnosis* of tinea is made by microscopical examination of scrapings from the lesions, which have been placed in 10 per cent potassium hydroxide.

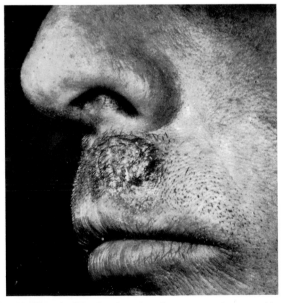

Fig. 30. Tinea barbae. Involvement of the moustache area with *T. discoides*, which responded well to griseofulvin.

Culture of the scales should also be done, as microscopy may sometimes fail to reveal the fungus. In ringworm of the scalp in children, hairs may fluoresce under Wood's light, depending on the species present. Wood's light is a mercury vapour lamp, containing cobalt and nickel oxide in a glass filter. Normal hair and skin fluoresce slightly under this light with a blue-white colour, but hairs infected with some types of ringworm fluoresce with a remarkable greenish colour (see Plate 24).

TREATMENT

The treatment of ringworm was revolutionized in 1959 by the introduction of griseofulvin. It is an antibiotic, and is obtained by the fermentation of several strains of penicillium.

It is effective against all known species of Trichophyton, Microsporum, and Epidermophyton.

It is *not* effective against *Candida albicans*, or any fungi causing systemic conditions.

Toxic reactions are rare; those reported include nausea, vomiting, headaches and urticaria. For contra-indications to griseofulvin therapy see page 34.

Resistance to the drug is also very rare.

Griseofulvin is taken by mouth. The average daily dose is 1·0 g daily, and the dose may all be taken at the same time after a meal; children's doses being measured according to weight and age (see p. 141). Griseofulvin is made up in tablets containing 125 or 500 mg in fine particles. Griseofulvin has superseded all other forms of treatment. When, however, only one or two lesions exist, a fungicidal ointment may be used. The exceptions to this rule are in cases of scalp infections when griseofulvin must always be used, and in cases caused by Trichophyton rubrum for which topical treatment is usually ineffective.

Prophylaxis in scalp infections consists in keeping the child away from school, and taking obvious measures at home to prevent spread to other children, so long as there is evidence of infection In the case of body, groin or foot infections, the patient should take care in only using a specified towel and bath mat, etc., although in schools and communal baths, where foot infections are not uncommon this is often impossible.

Tinea Pedis

Athlete's foot, ringworm of the feet

This condition is found mostly in young and middle-aged men, more commonly in summer than winter, and rarely in children. There are two types, namely an acute inflammatory, and a chronic dry type. The organism usually found in the acute type is *Trichophyton mentagrophytes*, and in the chronic type *Trichophyton rubrum*.

CLINICAL FEATURES

1. *Acute inflammatory*

This type arises from what has been for months or years a minimal infection, characterized by symptomless scaling in the toe-clefts, usually between the 4th and 5th toes. Suddenly an acute vesicular or vesiculo-pustular eruption begins which may spread over the feet and legs. Itching is common.

2. *Chronic dry*

This type is clinically mild, yet usually very difficult to cure. It is characterized by slight redness and scaling (Fig. 31), involving the soles, heels and sides of the feet (moccasin appearance). Acute exacerbations are uncommon. The nails invariably become involved, the changes being thickening under the nail, and friability of the nail.

DIAGNOSIS

Clinical signs of ringworm of the feet are not reliable and must be substantiated by microscopical examination of scrapings.

The condition must be differentiated from *contact dermatitis* caused by shoes, when the areas of contact with the shoes should correspond, *hyperidrosis*, which shows simple maceration between the toes, and in the chronic type of ringworm, from *psoriasis*, whose lesions show well-defined plaques.

TREATMENT

In the *acute* phase of the *acute type*, treat only with bland applications.

Complete or partial rest is very rewarding. Blisters should be opened, but not removed.

Potassium permanganate warm foot baths, 1 in 8,000 solution,

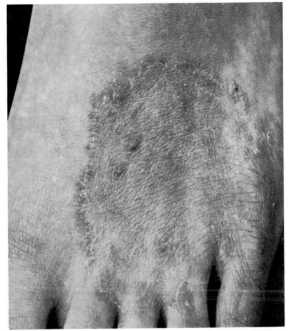

Fig. 31. Tinea pedis showing well-marked scaly edge and involvement of toe-clefts, particularly 4–5. Causative fungus, *T. mentagrophytes.*

should be given for 5 minutes two or three times a day until oozing has ceased. If skin has become too dry, apply hydrous emulsifying ointment B.P. Treatment with griseofulvin should also be started.

For the *chronic dry type*, apply Whitfield's ointment, Magenta paint B.P.C., or clotrimazole (Canesten) 1 per cent cream, and give griseofulvin 1·0 g daily for 3 weeks; however, results are often disappointing.

Tinea Manuum

Ringworm of the hands

As in ringworm of the feet, there are two clinical varieties, an acute

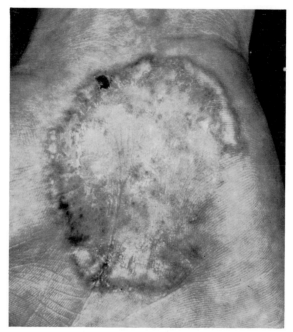

FIG. 32. Tinea manuum showing well-marked vesiculo-squamous edge from which fungi were demonstrated. Fungus, *T. mentagrophytes* (Institute of Dermatology, University of London).

and chronic, the acute being very uncommon in temperate climates. The fungi responsible for both varieties are invariably *Trichophyton rubrum*, or *T. mentagrophytes*.

CLINICAL FEATURES (Fig. 32)

These are similar to foot infection.

This condition hardly ever exists without coincidental involvement of the feet, and they should therefore always be examined, although the patient usually denies that there is anything wrong with them. Examination of the feet, in fact, should never be omitted when a rash exists on the hands.

DIAGNOSIS

This must be made by mycological investigation and from clinical signs regarded as corroborative rather than diagnostic evidence. Ringworm of the hands is not very common.

TREATMENT

This consists of giving 1 g of griseofulvin daily for 3 weeks, yet even after apparent cure has taken place, relapses occur in a notable percentage of cases. Fungicidal ointments may have to be used at the same time.

Tinea Unguium

Ringworm of the nails

The fungus commonly responsible for this condition is *Trichophyton rubrum. T. mentagrophytes, T. interdigitale, and E. floccosum* are much less common. Invariably ringworm of the feet is present.

CLINICAL FEATURES

Every degree of nail deformity may be seen, from one scarcely detectable to virtually complete disintegration of the nail plate (Fig. 33).

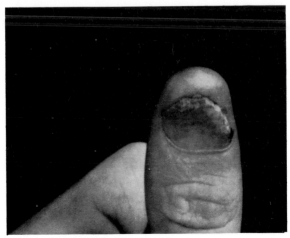

FIG. 33. Tinea of nail, *T. rubrum.*

The infection begins at the distal end of the nail plate and spreads proximally. The undersurface of the nail may be seen to be hyperkeratotic.

The colour of the nail does not alter unless bacterial invasion takes place, when it becomes greenish. Nevertheless, there is ordinarily a loss of the normal lustre of the nail.

DIAGNOSIS

This is made by microscopical and cultural examination of the nail clippings. The condition must be distinguished from *psoriasis*, which nearly always shows typical psoriatic lesions on the characteristic sites. *Dermatitis* of the fingers from any cause is liable to produce nail changes similar to fungus infection.

TREATMENT

Griseofulvin 1 g daily must be taken for many months before a cure is obtained; on an average 6 months for fingernails and 18 months for toenails. During this time the side-effects of griseofulvin must be considered; e.g. anaemia, and therefore regular blood counts must be performed. In some cases avulsion has also to be considered.

Cure of established toe-nail infection is difficult and rare.

Tinea Corporis; Tinea Circinata

Ringworm of the body

Practically all species of trichophyton and microsporum are capable of involving any area of smooth skin.

CAUSE

Microsporum canis, T. mentagrophytes, T. rubrum, and occasionally *T. tonsurans* and *T. verrucosum.*

Children are more susceptible than adults.

CLINICAL FEATURES

Four common varieties of lesions are seen, each usually being associated with a particular type of fungus.

The varieties are (1) annular, (2) plaque, (3) follicular, and (4) granulomatous.

1. The *annular type* produces red-ringed lesions, with tiny peri-

pheral vesicles, and a clear, slightly scaly centre. It may involve the scalp.

2. The *plaque type* is less inflammatory than the annular type, and may also involve the scalp. *T. tonsurans* is the usual organism found. Occasionally *T. rubrum* produces large plaques.

3. The *follicular* type shows a pustular folliculitis, usually of the neck, shoulders and arms, which may be quite painful. Granulomatous lesions sometimes occur. The source may be traced to pet white mice which may have been permitted to run up and down the arms of children. The organism is invariably *T. mentagrophytes*.

4. The *granulomatous type* is characterized by lesions looking like carbuncles. Suppuration is present and is due to the fungus, usually *T. verrucosum*, which also causes cattle ringworm, and can be transmitted from animal to patient. In this case, too, the scalp may be involved.

Other varieties exist, but they are all rare.

DIAGNOSIS

This is made by microscopy and culture when necessary. Wood's light is positive in some cases when the scalp is involved.

The disease must be distinguished from *pityriasis rosea*, in which no fungi are found, and where evolution is much more rapid. *Psoriasis* has heaped-up scales, nearly always on extensor surfaces, and vesicles are absent. *Eczema* shows no central clearing. *Seborrhoeic dermatitis* has greasy scales involving seborrhoeic areas, and where the lesion is not clear in the centre.

TREATMENT

Griseofulvin tablets are given, i.e. 1 g daily for 2–3 weeks, but if lesions number only one or two. Whitfield's ointment or clotrimazole (Canesten) 1 per cent cream, can be used instead.

Tinea Cruris

Ringworm of the Groin, Dhobie Itch

This condition occurs predominantly in males. It is usually spread by sharing bath towels, or is transferred from a co-existent foot infection. The organisms responsible are the same as those producing ringworm of the body. The condition is bilateral, but asymmetrical, and annular type lesions are produced (Plate 22). Itching may be quite marked.

In differential diagnosis, erythrasma (see page 120) must be considered.

TREATMENT

Griseofulvin is best. Topical therapy is messy and less effective.

Tinea Capitis

Ringworm of the scalp

This condition is characterized by scaly patches of different sizes in which are seen broken hairs. It occurs almost exclusively in children (Fig. 34, Plate 23).

CAUSE

Little of the anthropophilic variety is now seen in the British Isles. Animal types may be seen in country areas. *T. verrucosum* is still quite common. *M. canis* is rare.

CLINICAL FEATURES

The onset varies according to the fungus involved. Generally, however, it is gradual. The degree of inflammatory reaction in the patch also depends on the fungus present. If the condition is allowed to persist untreated, a folliculitis, or a carbuncular mass called a kerion, develops. As a result of modern methods of treatment, this is now rare.

The disease may spread to the eyelids, the neck and trunk, and these areas must be examined.

DIAGNOSIS

This is made by the clinical appearance of scaling and broken hairs, and microscopical examination of hairs in potassium hydroxide. Wood's light examination may also be useful (see p. 133 and Plate 24). In most cases of scalp ringworm, fluorescence occurs.

The condition must be differentiated from *seborrhoeic dermatitis* in which there are no broken hairs and greasy scales are present. *Alopecia areata* shows no scales, and the scalp is white, shiny and smooth.

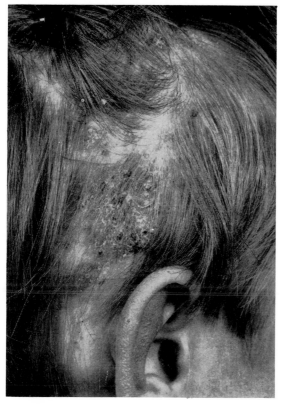

FIG. 34. Tinea capitis: causative fungus, *T. mentagrophytes* (Institute of Dermatology, University of London).

TREATMENT

Griseofulvin in a dosage of 25 mg per kg of body weight every second day for 2 weeks is usually effective when combined with local applications. A single dose of 3–4 g can also be curative.

For adults, 1·0 g daily for 3 weeks is adequate.

Whitfield's ointment should be applied daily to the affected areas, if only to prevent debris falling, and starch poultices may be required, when the lesions are blatantly pustular. Antibiotics are of no avail in pustular cases, as the purulent element is due to the toxic effects of the fungus and not bacteria.

Pityriasis Versicolor

Tinea Versicolor

This is a chronic, symptomless fungus infection due to *Malassezia furfur*, which appears in scales as hyphal elements and spores.

CLINICAL FEATURES

The onset is gradual. The lesions are macular and are fawn or café-au-lait. They are well defined, covered with fine branny scales, and they commonly affect the chest, back and axillae. Those affected usually wear woollens, often sleep in them, and bath seldom.

DIAGNOSIS

This is made by finding the fungus in scales. The infection must be distinguished from vitiligo, chloasma, and other pigmentary disorders.

TREATMENT

Frequent washing and change of underclothes which should be cotton. Apply clotrimazole cream (Canesten) or miconazole cream (Dermonistat) b.d. for two weeks. Alternatively, a 2·5 selenium sulphide suspension (Selsun), applied generously and left on overnight, may be used. Following treatment, the finger nails should be scrubbed to prevent development of a latent source of infection.

Candidiasis

Moniliasis, thrush, oidiomycosis

Candidiasis is caused by a yeast-like fungus, *Candida albicans*, and produces a variety of lesions of the skin and mucous membranes.

PREDISPOSING FACTORS

Occupation: housewives, bartenders and bakers are prone to develop paronychia. Excessive immersion in water allows the organism to enter below the softened nail-fold.

Other illnesses: Debilitating diseases, alcoholism, diabetes, hyperidrosis and obesity may predispose to candida infection.

CLINICAL FEATURES

Localized types

(1) Onychia and paronychia. These conditions are characterized by bolstering of the affected nail-fold from which, perhaps, a bead of pus may be expressed with gentle pressure. The nail is usually ridged as a result of the disease, and a dirty greenish-brown discoloration of the lateral aspects of the nail takes place.

(2) Intertrigo. This is characterized by well-defined red, moist patches with a scalloped edge, commonly in the submammary folds, groins, umbilicus, axillae, or intergluteal folds (Plate 25). Intertrigo is also found in obese patients in the above-mentioned areas without evidence of candida; sweating causes maceration and gives a clinical impression of candida.

(3) Perlèche. See chapter 18.

(4) Intra-oral thrush. This is seen as a whitish loose membrane on the inner surface of the cheeks, or on the palate of babies, children or young adults.

(5) Superficial glossitis. This may appear in adults as a beefy-red, smooth tongue.

(6) Vaginitis, vulval ulcers, and balanoposthitis.

Generalized types

These may be cutaneous or systemic, but are uncommon.

DIAGNOSIS

This can be made by finding the organism in scrapings from lesions.

TREATMENT

Prophylaxis is difficult, and includes attention to any predisposing cause. For paronychia, use finger stalls or rubber gloves when washing.

In cases of paronychia, use Nystan ointment, or amphotericin-B lotion (Fungilin), t.d.s., by inserting the application under the nail-fold with a flat orange-stick. Clotrimazole cream (Canesten), miconazole cream (Dermonistat) or Eusol are also useful. Paronychia may take 6–10 weeks to clear with any of these forms of treatment.

For intertrigo, use Nystan ointment or Fungilin lotion, t.d.s. In non-candidal cases, a dusting powder, e.g. Zeasorb or a steroid cream will reduce the inflammation invariably present.

For oral thrush, use Nystan suspension (nystatin 100,000 i.u. per ml) q.d.s. with nystan tablets, one q.d.s.

CHAPTER 11

Diseases due to Viruses

Warts: Herpes zoster: Herpes simplex: Kaposi's Varicelliform Eruption: Molluscum Contagiosum: Chicken Pox: Smallpox: Measles: German Measles: Vaccinia: Orf

Introduction

Viruses are very minute organisms, smaller than bacteria and not visible by the usual microscopic examination. They cannot carry on a free life of their own like bacteria, and live intracellularly, breeding and multiplying in living cells.

They tend to have certain fixed habits, which are useful for identification purposes. They usually focus their attention on one particular kind of host and one particular kind of tissue and produce in that tissue particular types of intra-cellular inclusion bodies.

The diseases which are described below are considered to be viral in origin, and this is substantiated by the distinctive inclusion bodies which can be found when the tissue has been appropriately stained.

In herpes zoster and simplex they are called Lipschütz bodies, in molluscum contagiosum, molluscum bodies, in varicella and variola, Guarnieri bodies. All diseases due to viruses are infectious or contagious, though some more mildly so than others.

Warts

Nearly all warts, or verrucae, are of the common type and are viral in origin. Other less common varieties are (1) syphilitic, (2) malignant and (3) tuberculous which are dealt with elsewhere.

Common warts are the bane of the dermatologist's practice. They may form a third of hospital cases, they are by no means straightforward to treat successfully when large numbers are present, and are liable to recur. They also appear on new areas following eradication of existing lesions. Some individuals are more susceptible than others,

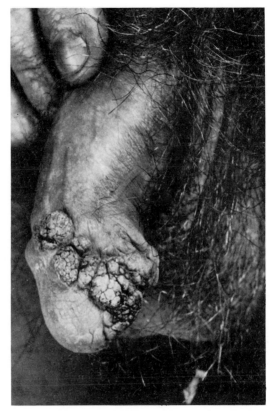

Fig. 35. Penile warts (Institute of Dermatology, University of London).

including the author, and it is noticeable that in a household or in a school, where contacts are closer than normal, many remain immune to this infection—a characteristic of virus diseases.

Warts are well-defined tumours of varying size, having a rounded or pointed top and a sessile or pedunculated base. There are several clinical forms of the common wart: (1) the common, (2) the plantar, (3) the plane or juvenile, (4) the filiform, (5) the acuminate.

PATHOLOGY

Hyperkeratosis, acanthosis, and papillomatosis are the principal changes seen in warts, and these hypertrophic reactions account for the density of warts. Inclusion bodies are present in some, but not all warts.

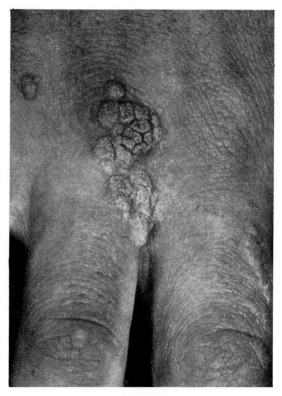

Fig. 36. Common warts.

CLINICAL FEATURES

(1) *The common wart* (*Verruca vulgaris*)
Lesions are pin-head to pea-size. Sites: hands and fingers chiefly
(Fig. 36).

(2) *The plantar wart* (*Verruca plantaris*)
is pea-sized or larger and may resemble a corn (Figs. 37, 38). Pressure
points on the plantar surface of the foot are chiefly affected, but no
part is exempt.

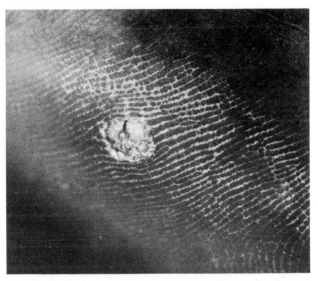

Fɪɢ. 37. Plantar wart of ten years' duration, having weathered many
different local applications, and some operative procedures.

(3) *The plane wart* (*Verruca plana*)
so-called because they are flat-topped. They are very discrete and
flesh-coloured and, if single, may be difficult to observe. Sites: the
face, forehead, the backs of the hands and the front of the knees are
most commonly attacked. Young people are predominantly affected.

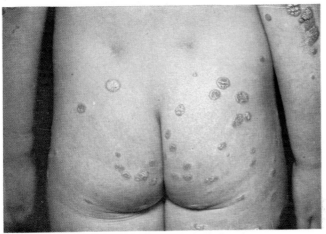

PLATE 1. Psoriasis (Dr G. A. Hodgson).

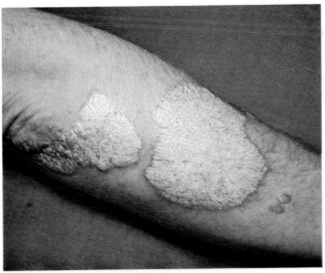

PLATE 2a. Psoriasis (Dr G. A. Hodgson).

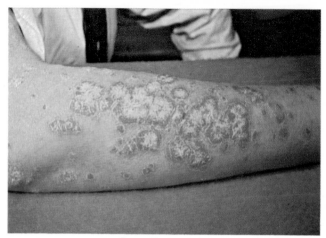

PLATE 2b. Psoriasis.

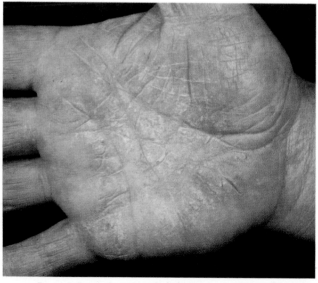

PLATE 3. Psoriasis: palmar lesions (Dr G. A. Hodgson).

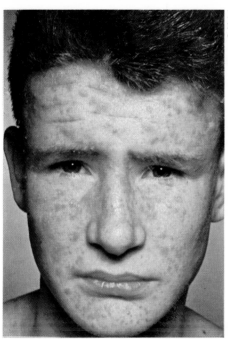

PLATE 4. Psoriasis: facial lesions (Dr G. A. Hodgson).

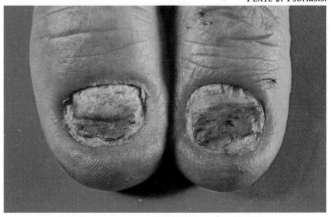

PLATE 5. Psoriasis.

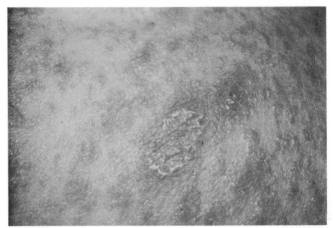

PLATE 6. Pityriasis rosea, showing the salmon-rose colour of the condition

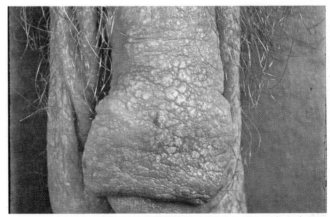

PLATE 7. Lichen planus. Violaceous, shiny, slightly scaly, penile lesions (Skin Department, London Hospital).

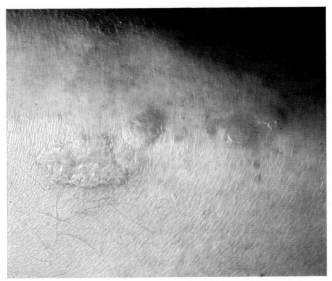

PLATE 8. Lichen planus. Violaceous, scaly, shiny lesions on the forearm (Dr G. A. Hodgson).

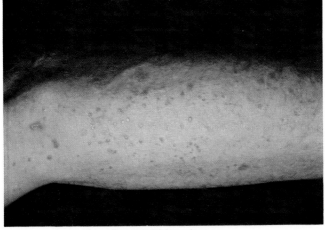

PLATE 9. Lichen planus.

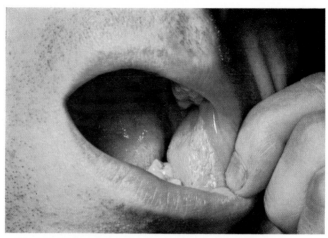

PLATE 10. Lichen planus, showing white patches on the buccal mucosa, and more discrete lesions on the tongue (Dr G. A. Hodgson).

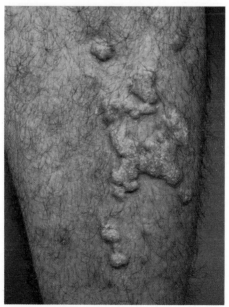

PLATE 11. Lichen planus, showing lesions of the hypertrophic variety.

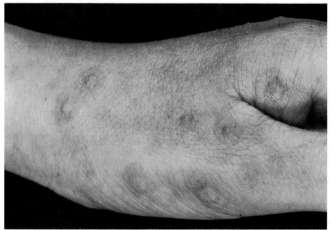

PLATE 12. Erythema multiforme showing iris-like lesions (Institute of Dermatology, University of London).

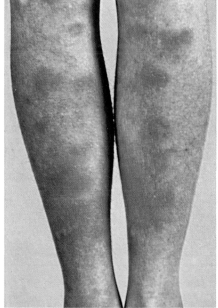

PLATE 13. Erythema nodosum. Bright-red, smooth lesions, in this case associated with acute follicullar tonsilitus.

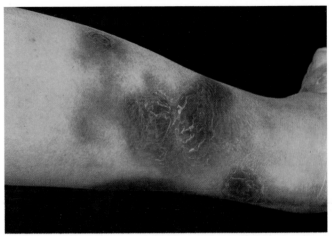

PLATE 14. Erythema induratum (Institute of Dermatology, University of London).

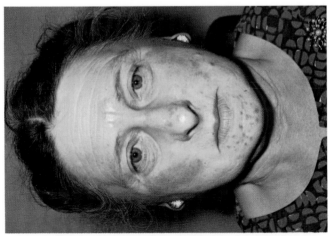

PLATE 15. Rosacea showing butterfly distribution on cheeks and nose, with pustules on left side of face and chin. The more intense redness of the cheeks is due to excessive application of flourinated steroids.

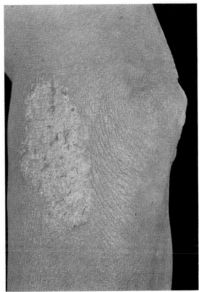

PLATE 16. Localized neurodermatitis. Well-defined chronic lesion showing superficial adherent and uneven scaling, with some crusting (Institute of Dermatology, University of London).

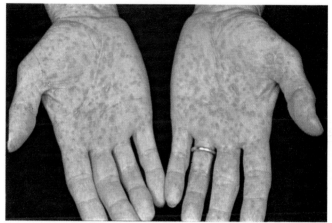
PLATE 17. Secondary syphilide: papulo-squamous lesions.

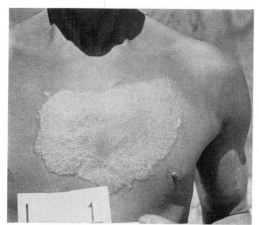

PLATE 18. Tuberculoid leprosy (Dr D. G. Jamison). Single anaesthetic lesion, A.F.B. absent.

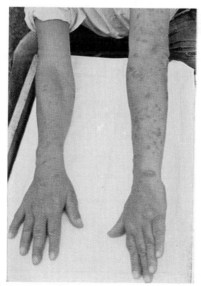

PLATE 19. Lepromatous leprosy (Dr W. H. Jopling). Multiple small lesions which are not anaesthetic. Similar lesions on face, trunk and legs. A.F.B. very numerous.

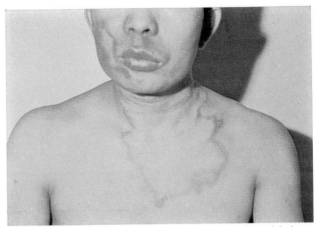

PLATE 20. Borderline leprosy (Dr W. H. Jopling). Several lesions, all showing moderate anaesthesia. A.F.B. scanty. Note left-sided facial palsy.

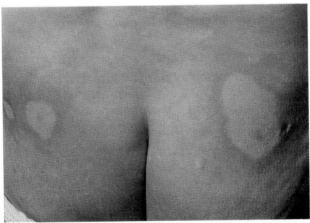

PLATE 21. Borderline leprosy (Dr W. H. Jopling). Several lesions, all showing slight anaesthesia. A.F.B. in moderate numbers.

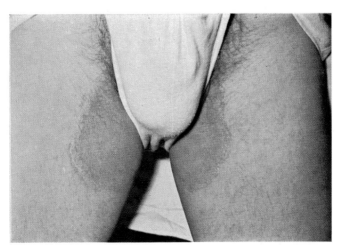

PLATE 22. Tinea cruris. Well-defined lesions with a scaly edge (Skin Department, London Hospital).

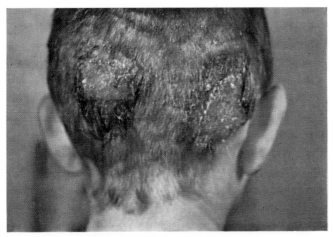

PLATE 23. Tinea capitis (*T. discoides*) (Dr Martin Beare).

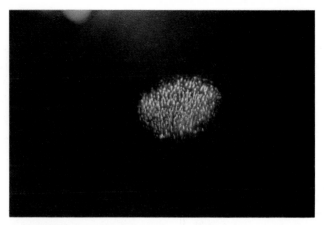

PLATE 24. Tinea capitis fluorescing under Wood's light (Institute of Dermatology, University of London).

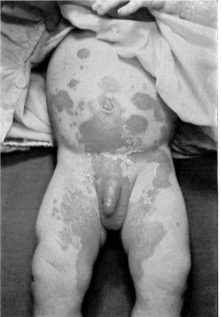

PLATE 25. Candidiasis. Polycyclic borders fringed by white epidermis (Dr Martin Beare).

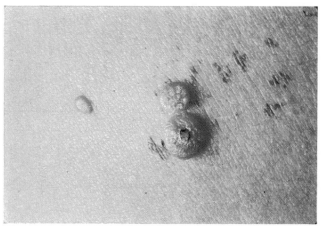

PLATE 26. Molluscum contagiosum. Pearly lesions on the back, showing the central depression from which a caseous plug may be squeezed.

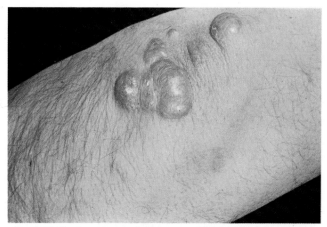

PLATE 27. Xanthomatous nodules in man with raised blood cholesterol (Institute of Dermatology, University of London).

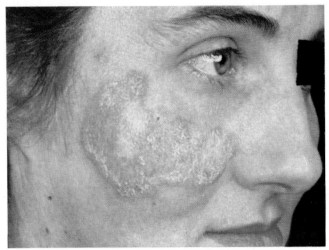

PLATE 28. Lupus erythematosus: chronic variety (Institute of Dermatology, University of London).

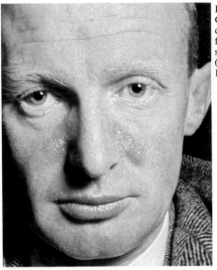

PLATE 29. Lupus erythematosu Chronic variety, showing well-demarcated scaly lesions on the face and left eyebrow, simulating seborrhoeic dermati (Skin Department, London Hospital).

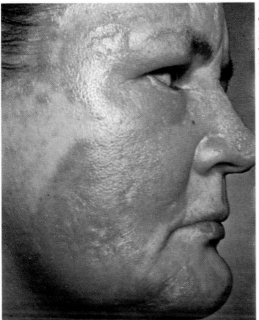

PLATE 30. Lupus erythematosus. Diffuse erythema of the face, in a case with systemic involvement (Dr G. A. Hodgson).

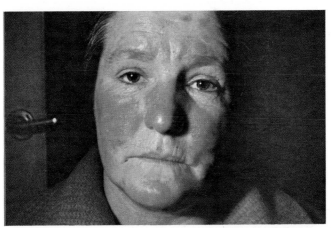

PLATE 31. Sarcoid, in this case simulating rosacea (Dr Martin Beare).

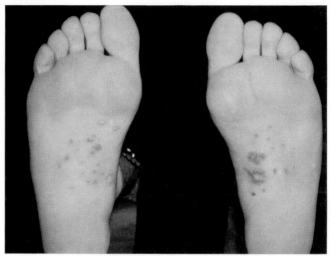

PLATE 32. Reiter's disease showing characteristic vesico-pustules.

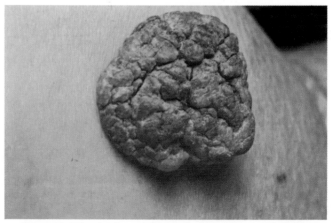

PLATE 33. Seborrhoeic wart. Unusually large lesion on the back.

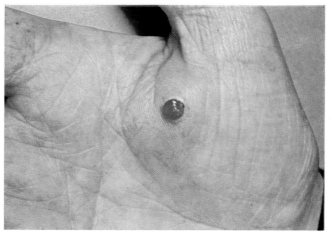

PLATE 34. Granuloma pyogenicum (Dr Martin Beare).

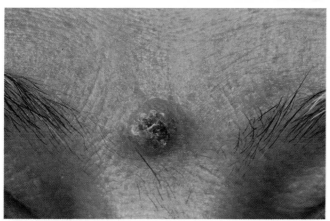

PLATE 35. Kerato-acanthoma: well-developed lesion with central crater
(Institute of Dermatology, University of London).

PLATE 36. Paget's disease of the nipple, indurated and infiltrated with destruction of the nipple.

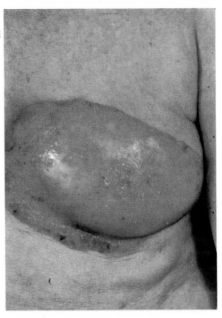

PLATE 37. Haemangioma (Institute of Dermatology, University of London).

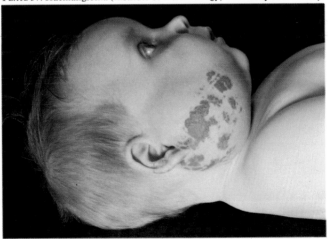

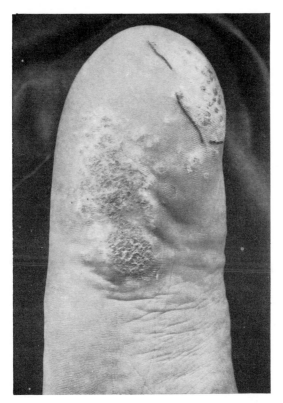

Fig. 38. Plantar warts, mosaic variety.

(4) *The filiform wart* (*Verruca filiformis*)
is pedunculated and may be as thick as a match and up to a quarter
of an inch long. It is commonly seen on the necks of middle-aged
women and the bearded area of men.

(5) *The acuminate wart* (*Condylomata acuminata*)
is soft and fleshy and resembles a miniature cauliflower; with time they vegetate and stink. They develop on mucocutaneous areas, especially the ano-genital.

TREATMENT

There is no specific treatment for warts. Any form of conservative or radical treatment may succeed or fail. One physician will succeed with an identical treatment with which a colleague has failed. Such is the fickle nature of warts. A number of warts, probably 5 per cent, disappear spontaneously, and many can be tempted to leave their host by remedies as varied as the application of early morning spittle, the eye of a potato or sticking-plaster, providing the practitioner can convince the patient of their value.

Common warts
40 per cent salicylic acid in collodion, or 5 per cent picric acid may be applied daily. Cauterization under local anaesthetic or curettage is the most effective treatment and most useful when few warts are present. The application of liquid nitrogen or oxygen is an impressive form of therapy, but painful and not always effective.

Plane warts
may respond to local applications, such as 2 per cent salicylic acid in spirit. No matter what treatment is used, these warts may disappear overnight.

Plantar warts
Are best treated by cautery or curettage. Otherwise formaldehyde 1 per cent in water applied daily for 5 minutes on cotton wool may be curative after 4–8 weeks. The mosaic variety may be treated by weekly applications of 40 per cent salicylic acid plasters, kept in position by sticking plaster. The plaster must be carefully applied to the wart, avoiding the surrounding skin as much as possible. Otherwise painful desquamation will occur. Posafilin ointment carefully applied at night may also be used, but can cause some discomfort.

Filiform warts
Are easily cauterized.

Acuminate warts
usually respond to 2–5 per cent podophyllin in alcohol or tinct. benz. co. applied carefully every 2 or 3 days for 3 or 4 applications. If the application is placed on normal skin, it causes a painful burn. If it fails, cautery is the treatment of choice.

PROGNOSIS
Recurrences are by no means uncommon. The acuminate wart has been reported, very occasionally, as capable of malignant change.

Herpes Zoster

Shingles

This is an acute infection of nerve structures producing groups of vesicles distributed along the course of one or more peripheral nerves on one side of the body. The inflammatory changes are usually confined to one posterior root ganglion.

CAUSE
The virus is either identical with or closely related to the virus of chicken-pox, since it is not uncommon for healthy contacts with either disease to contract the other.

Age
Any age may be affected, but it occurs chiefly in adults.

Season
As in so many viral diseases, infection is more likely during the spring and autumn.

Secondary to other conditions
Less commonly the eruption appears following trauma, pressure from vertebral tumours, or the enlarged glands of Hodgkin's disease or leukaemia, or infections such as meningitis.

PATHOLOGY
The vesicle is intra-epidermal and is produced by the degeneration of epidermal and blood cells and fibrin, which it then contains.

The epidermal cells are apparently inflated, appearing as balloons. They stain poorly, and may be un-nucleated, or contain many nuclei. In the basophilic nuclei of the balloon cells are found the eosinophilic Lipschütz inclusion bodies, and the epithelial cells of the hair follicles and sebaceous glands may be similarly affected.

Another notable change is reticular degeneration, which means cavity formation in the epidermis, resulting in multilocular vesicles. Reticular degeneration, it must be remembered, occurs sometimes in dermatitis. The dermis shows generalized vascular dilatation, a polymorphic and lymphocytic infiltrate, and oedema in the upper third of the dermis.

The posterior nerve root ganglia show interstitial inflammation, and degenerative changes.

CLINICAL FEATURES

Pain of varying degrees of severity in the distribution of the root or roots affected precedes the vesicular eruption by a day or two. In the appendix area, for example, the pain may cause considerable difficulty in diagnosis before the rash appears. Mild pyrexia and fairly severe irritation may also occur.

The lesions are vesicular containing clear fluid and develop from papules. After a few days, the vesicles rupture and crusted lesions form. Occasionally the lesions are pustular or haemorrhagic. Their size is tiny or pea-sized. The site may be anywhere on the body and the distribution is nearly always unilateral (Fig. 39).

Other varieties

(1) Ophthalmic or Gasserian herpes involving the 1st division of the Vth cranial nerve is always serious, leading sometimes to keratitis or blindness.

(2) Geniculate herpes (the Ramsay-Hunt syndrome) commences with tonsillar or ear pain, and is followed by a vesicular eruption on the pinna, external ear, or fauces, loss of taste of the anterior two-thirds of the tongue, and may produce a facial palsy of lower motor neurone type.

Complications

Post-herpetic neuralgia occurs especially in old people, and may be

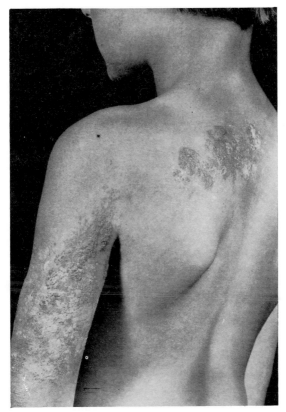

Fig. 39. Herpes zoster showing vesicular and unilateral eruption (Institute of Dermatology, University of London).

so distressing and chronic as to induce suicidal depression. It may, however, clear spontaneously in a few months.

DIAGNOSIS

This is made by the history, the grouping of painful vesicles, and the unilateral distribution. *Herpes simplex* is sometimes bilateral and commonly recurrent, but the first attack may be difficult to distinguish from zoster.

TREATMENT

There is nothing specific. Rest is paramount for the elderly.

Aspirin or phenacetin orally may be given for pain and, when intense, morphia injections. A steroid spray combined with an antibiotic (e.g. Terra-Cortril) will control both irritation and secondary infection.

External

Calamine lotion, or a steroid lotion with an antibiotic should be dabbed on 3 or 4 times daily. The lesions should be protected from trauma with gauze.

Internal

Aspirin may be given to relieve pain, whilst steroids may help in shortening the period of discomfort and reducing the risk of neuralgia, which can occur in old people.

Post-herpetic neuralgia usually offers a great challenge to ingenuity. Radiant heat to the healed area, X-ray to the affected ganglia, morphia, and steroids by mouth are some of the therapies which may be tried.

PROGNOSIS

This is better for young people than for old. Second attacks are uncommon.

Herpes Simplex

This is an acute disorder characterized by grouped vesicles on a red base, usually affecting the lips, face, or genitalia. The condition may be recurrent or non-recurrent, the former type being the rule. This disease presents a different picture from herpes zoster.

The word simplex in the title is extremely misleading, as the secondary type is notably recurrent, despite treatment.

CAUSE

The common oral lesions are caused by Herpes simplex virus Type 1 strains, the genital lesions by Type 2. These strains can usually be identified in the laboratory although it is not yet a routine procedure. Either strain can be grown from swabs taken from lesions, and placed in either Hansen's virus transport, or Stuart's transport medium.

There is a lot of clinical serological and epidermiological evidence to show that HSV2 strains are nearly always sexually transmitted as a result of oro-genital intercourse.

Predisposing factors may be strong sunlight, fevers, gastro-intestinal upsets, or emotional stress, in some cases.

PATHOLOGY
This is similar to zoster.

CLINICAL FEATURES
Recurrent type. Unlike zoster, there is only slight discomfort when the lesions appear, the onset being sudden.

Lesions are vesicular at first, later rupturing and forming crusted lesions. Sites involved are chiefly the lips, face, the genitalia and trunk. Lesions are grouped, as all herpetic lesions are, but differ from zoster in that they are sometimes bilateral.

In female genital herpes, there is a tendency for urethral involvement by vesicles which can lead to painful micturition and, occasionally, acute retention. Cervicitis, which may be severe, is not infrequent, and the cervix should always be examined in cases of vulval herpes.

COMPLICATIONS
Some evidence exists showing an association between genital HSV2 infections and carcinoma of the cervix. The precise nature and significance of this relationship is not yet clear, but many authorities consider that all women who have had such infections should have a prolonged cytological follow-up.

COURSE
The lesions clear up in one or two weeks but are liable to recur, and when they do so, always attack the same area as before.

Other varieties
The non-recurrent type is seen in children between 6 months and

7 years of age. Pyrexia may reach 104°F (40°C). A large vesicle appears in the mouth, breaks down into an ulcer, and heals within a fortnight.

DIAGNOSIS

Herpes simplex must be distinguished from herpes zoster. The possibility of syphilis as an alternative or additional diagnosis should be remembered.

TREATMENT

Idoxuridine 10 per cent in dimethyl sulphoxide (DMSO) applied q.d.s. is only useful during the first 3 days of the attack. Otherwise, pHisoHex lotion will keep lesions clean. Oxytetracycline ointments are usually prescribed if the lesion becomes infected. A small dose of X-rays may shorten an attack, and lengthen the interval before the next one.

Kaposi's Varicelliform Eruption

Eczema herpeticum

This is an acute, contagious, vesicular, febrile eruption, caused by the herpes simplex or vaccinia virus, superimposed on eczematous skin. It occurs predominantly in male infants and children.

CLINICAL FEATURES

The onset is sudden. Lesions are vesicular, occurring in crops on eczematous skin, which becomes oedematous. The attacks last 10–14 days.

DIAGNOSIS

is made by history of exposure to herpes simplex and the identification of Lipschütz inclusion bodies in early vesicles.

TREATMENT

Isolation, and antibiotics to counteract secondary infection.

PROGNOSIS

In severe cases, death may occur.

Molluscum Contagiosum

This disorder is characterized by rounded molluscous or shell-like lesions, showing on close examination an apical depression.

CAUSE

A virus, both auto-inoculable and contagious. It can be transmitted by the contacts of everyday life, and during sexual intercourse.

Predisposing factors
Age. Infants and children are most commonly affected.

Occupation. This disorder is not uncommon in beauty specialists and masseurs who contract it from their clients, and also transmit it to them.

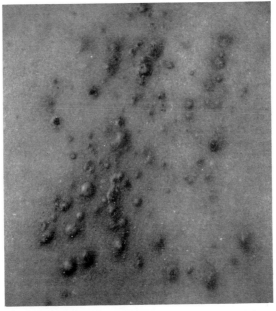

FIG. 40. Molluscum contagiosum. Pearly papules and nodules with some typically umbilicated.

PATHOLOGY

The epidermis develops into large pear-shaped lobules, extending itself into the dermis. Many epidermal cells degenerate and desquamate, and because of this, a cavity forms on the surface producing what is seen clinically as a central depression.

CLINICAL FEATURES

The incubation period is not exactly known. There are no symptoms. The onset is gradual. The lesions are papular at first, later becoming nodular (Fig. 40). Their size varies from pin-point to pin-head, and they are slow to develop. Their shape is slightly pointed or globular at first, later becoming flattened on the top, the surface being umbilicated. Their colour is pink or pearly (Plate 26) and they are shiny. Sites commonly involved are the face, eyelids, and genitalia, but no area is exempt. The number of lesions may vary from one or two to thirty or more. The contents of these lesions consists of a thick yellowish curdy substance.

Conjuctivitis may occur with eye-lid lesions, whilst some develop eczema around them, a few weeks after the onset. Both conditions clear up, following treatment of the lesions.

COURSE

Untreated, the lesions persist for many months; sometimes some of them dry up spontaneously.

DIAGNOSIS

Once seen, the discrete, pearly, shiny, umbilicated lesions are unmistakable.

TREATMENT

Lift off the crusted top, or incise the top of the lesion and express or curette the curdy contents. Then insert an orange-stick impregnated with iodine for a few seconds or 1 per cent cantharidin in equal parts of water and acetone.

Chicken-Pox

Varicella

This acute infectious disease is characterized by crops of bright red vesicles, caused by a virus identical, or closely allied to, the virus of herpes zoster. It is most infectious in the early stages, but also infectious, though less so, while crusts remain.

CLINICAL FEATURES

Prodromal malaise may or may not occur. Pyrexia is usual, varying between 99°–101°F (37·2°–38·3°C).

Lesions appear on the first or second day. First of all papular, they soon become vesicular, and later pustular. Scars often follow resolution. Sites commonly affected are the trunk and face. The rash, unlike smallpox, is most profuse on the trunk, and sparsest at the periphery of the limbs. The mouth and throat also become affected. Duration of the disease is 3–7 days.

TREATMENT

is symptomatic. Calamine lotion is helpful for itching.

Smallpox

Variola

This is an acute infectious and contagious fever, characterized by macules, papules, vesicles, pustules, crusts and scarring, with constitutional symptoms of varying severity.

Quite often, during epidemics, the dermatologist is asked to confirm a diagnosis of smallpox. Since vaccination is not compulsory the risk of epidemics is still considerable, and it is, therefore, as important as ever to be familiar with the different facets of the disease.

There are three varieties of the virus causing smallpox:

1. Asiatic smallpox (variola major), which has a high mortality rate.
2. Variola minor, which causes a far milder disease.
3. The third is used for vaccination, which cannot cause a serious disease.

No infant with eczema should be vaccinated against smallpox (see p. 42).

PATHOLOGY

Numerous Guarnieri bodies are found in the early stages. They are eosinophilic, round or oval, and are surrounded by a notably clear halo. Reticular degeneration is well marked, but unlike herpes zoster there are few balloon cells.

CLINICAL FEATURES

The incubation period of 12 days (in most patients) is followed suddenly by severe headache, pyrexia 103°–104°F (39·4°–40°C), pain in the back, rigors, and generalized aching of the limbs. A day or two after the appearance of the rash the temperature subsides, and the patient improves. This is a period when optimism is dangerous, for a few days later, as pustular lesions develop, the fever returns in full spate, and the patient becomes gravely ill again. If the patient recovers, the temperature slowly subsides again as the pustules dry up.

Prodromal purpuric lesions are seen in severe cases from the start. Lesions characteristic of smallpox appear on the third day as macules; within 24 hours they become papular, about three days later they become vesicular, and a few days afterwards, pustular. Three or four days later, crusts form, and in several weeks' time the crusts fall off. The sequence is therefore:

Macules—Papules—Vesicles—Pustules—Crusts.

All the lesions pass through this series of changes at the same time.

Sites first affected are the hands, wrists, forehead and mouth, mucosal lesions often being very severe. The rash spreads from the outer parts of the body towards the trunk, contrariwise to chicken-pox.

Complications

include broncho-pneumonia, conjunctivitis, otitis media, corneal ulceration with subsequent opacities, encephalitis and cardiac failure.

DIAGNOSIS

Sometimes difficult in mild cases to distinguish from chicken-pox. In chicken-pox there is far more involvement of the trunk, and the lesions appear in crops. Smallpox can be diagnosed with certainty by finding Guarnieri bodies in fluid from vesicles.

TREATMENT

There is no specific therapy. Skilled nursing is of the greatest importance. Aureomycin by mouth eliminates secondary infection.

Recently, trials with N-methylisatin P-thiosemicarbazone (Marboran) in the prophylaxis of smallpox have proved this drug to be invaluable in its prophylactic effect, regardless of the vaccination status of contacts.

Measles

This is an acute infectious and contagious disease, characterized by a macular rash, coryza, and upper respiratory catarrh.

Infection in the first 3 months of life is impossible, as a result of passive immunity conferred by the mother, but at any time afterwards the individual becomes highly susceptible. Transmission is by direct contact, from the nose, mouth, or respiratory tract. Infectivity lasts for 2 weeks after onset of the rash.

CLINICAL FEATURES

10–14 days after exposure, coryza, cough, and fever set in. The rash is always itchy.

Koplik's spots are diagnostic, and are visible on the first day. Koplik's spots are tiny white papules, like grains of salt, best seen on the mucous membrane of the cheeks opposite the molars.

On the 4th day, a pink macular rash which first appears behind the ears spreads over the face, trunk and limbs. The macules are small, being about 3–5 mm in diameter, but they coalesce into large irregular areas as the disease progresses, and finally fade as pale scaling lesions.

Complications

are principally due to secondary infection, resulting in bronchopneumonia, or otitis media.

DIAGNOSIS

Distinguish from German measles, which is much milder, and has no prodromal symptoms.

TREATMENT

Bed rest until the temperature has been normal for a week. Oxy-tetraclines should be given to prevent bacterial complications.

German Measles

Rubella

This is a mild infectious disease, characterized by a macular rash. When contracted by women in the first four months of a pregnancy, it often leads to developmental defects in the foetus. However, rubella antibody tests are now part of routine ante-natal care and the frequency of these defects should fall. Transmission is by direct contact. Infectivity exists at all stages of the disease. Incubation period, 14–21 days.

CLINICAL FEATURES

Lesions are macular. Sites first affected—scalp and face, followed by a general spread, lasting 1–3 days. Occipital glands become enlarged and tender.

TREATMENT

is rarely required.

Vaccinia

Cowpox

This is an eruptive disease occurring chiefly in the cow, but also produced in man by auto-inoculation or, very rarely, as a general infection.

One or more lesions occur on the body 7–14 days after vaccination. Ocular palsy and encephalitis are rare features of the disease.

Eczema vaccinatum describes vaccinia superimposed on eczema (see page 42).

Orf

This produces a contagious, pustular dermatitis in sheep or goats, and is contracted by those handling infected animals dead or alive.

The incubation period of 3–7 days is followed by the appearance of a firm, painless, dark papule which enlarges to form a domed pustule which may contain a little serum or blood, but mainly granulation tissue. Lesions are usually single, and commonly found on the fingers and hands. The condition is self-limiting, clearing in 4–8 weeks. Mild local remedies are sometimes required.

CHAPTER 12

Bullous Diseases

Dermatitis Herpetiformis: Pemphigus: Pemphigoid

Bullous disorders are not common and may be congenital or acquired.

The most important *congenital* form is epidermolysis bullosa, of which there are two varieties: a simple and a dystrophic type, the latter being characterized by lesions healing with severe scarring. A very rare lethal form also exists.

The most important *acquired* varieties of bullous eruptions are:

1. Dermatitis herpetiformis.
2. Pemphigus.
3. Pemphigoid.

Dermatitis Herpetiformis

This is a chronic condition characterized by macules, papules, vesicles and bullae, surrounded by erythema, which, as herpetiform suggests, results in the lesions usually being grouped as they are in herpes zoster. Another factor of much more importance to the patient is the burning and itching which varies in severity and always accompanies the condition.

The cause is not known. Both sexes are affected at all ages, but chiefly adult males.

PATHOLOGY

The bullae and vesicles form below the epidermis, unlike pemphigus. An important feature whose absence or presence must be noted is that of acantholysis (see p. 11), which is absent in this disorder, and present in pemphigus. An eosinophilic infiltrate is another major sign, being obvious in the bullae and around blood vessels.

CLINICAL FEATURES

The onset is commonly gradual with macules and papules. Vesicles and bullae develop, which are tense and clear at first, but later become cloudy. The groups of lesions have irregular patterns, and excoriations from scratching are notable. The sites usually affected are the forearms and thighs, scapular and lumbosacral areas, while the distribution of the rash is symmetrical. Oral mucosa is attacked at times. Diarrhoea may be present in some cases, and a barium meal may show changes associated with malabsorption. The significance of this correlation is as yet not clear.

Laboratory aids

The blood eosinophilia is high, being between 10 and 30 per cent.

COURSE

It is typical of this disease to come and go, the intervals of relapse and remission varying between weeks and months, for up to 10 or 15 years, and very occasionally longer.

Other varieties

A juvenile type of dermatitis herpetiformis exists, which may start at infancy, and usually resolves at puberty.

TREATMENT

External

Calamine lotion, or a steroid lotion to alleviate symptoms slightly.

Internal

Diamino-diphenyl-sulphone (dapsone) is the drug of choice. 100 mg tablets twice a day for 2 weeks, followed by 100 mg daily or less; if less controls the disease, it is given as long as is necessary. Iron should be given at the same time to offset any tendency to a normocytic anaemia, which the drug may provoke.

Sulphapyridine, 0·5–1 g daily, has a similar effect, but may produce disturbing toxic effects. Steroids are of little help.

A gluten-free diet should always be tried as about 70 per cent of patients have a gluten-sensitive enteropathy, essentially similar to that of coeliac disease.

DIAGNOSIS

This is made by the itching, the grouping of the lesions, and their multiformity. For differential diagnosis, see end of this chapter.

Pemphigus

This is a chronic disorder characterized by recurrent bullae of the skin, and/or mucous membranes. Two types of pemphigus exist: (1) pemphigus vulgaris, (2) pemphigus foliaceus. Each has a variant, namely, P. vegetans and P. erythematosus. P. vulgaris only will be dealt with here. The other three varieties are relatively rare.

Before the introduction of steroid treatment it was fatal within a few months or years of its onset. The cause is not established, although present knowledge indicates that it may be one of the auto-immune diseases. It is not infectious or contagious. The sexes are equally affected, and it is a disease of middle age.

PATHOLOGY

The bullae form in the epidermis, in contrast to dermatitis herpetiformis, owing to degeneration and liquefaction of the epidermal cells. Acantholysis, in fact, is present. In scrapings from the floor of a fresh bulla, the degenerated cells can be easily found. They are round, and contain spherical nuclei. The cytoplasm of the cell is markedly clear, except for the edge of the cell, which appears as a definite dark blue ring.

CLINICAL FEATURES

The onset is insidious. The bullae are at first tense, round, and contain serum, which soon becomes purulent as the bullae become flaccid. The skin around the bullae is normal. The bullae soon rupture, and whether in the mouth or on the skin leave raw areas (Fig. 41), which are extremely tender, when crusts form. Their size varies, they can be as big as a plum, and any site may be involved. The oral lesions are often the first signs of the disease.

The patient's general condition deteriorates rapidly in accordance with the severity of the skin lesions.

Nikolsky's sign is invariably present. This means that when firm pressure with the finger is exerted on normal skin, the epidermis slides off owing to its generally poor attachment to the underlying

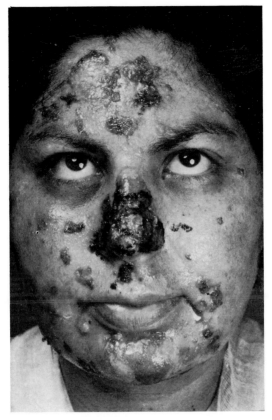

FIG. 41. Pemphigus. 3 years' duration, with remissions (Skin Department, London Hospital).

dermis. This sign may be elicited in other severe bullous eruptions, such as those due to dermatitis herpetiformis, epidermolysis bullosa, or drugs.

Eosinophilia and leucocytosis sometimes occur. The lesions occur in waves, and sometimes quite long periods of remission occur.

DIAGNOSIS

This is made by the character of the bullae and acantholysis. At the onset it is difficult, without a period of observation, to differentiate it from other conditions it imitates.

For differentiation, see table at the end of this chapter.

TREATMENT

Steroids and/or methotrexate (see p. 35) can save the life of these patients, although death can occur in spite of treatment. For some authorities, methotrexate is the treatment of choice in this condition, and also in pemphigoid (see below).

Methotrexate is given when prednisolone has brought the condition under control, or alternatively, 10 mg methotrexate twice a week for varying periods up to 6 months can be given in conjunction with steroids, before reducing the steroid dosage. Methotrexate appears not to influence mucosal lesions, for which triamcinolone in orabase can be applied.

The dangers of methotrexate are not much more than those of giving huge doses of steroids, both of which of course should be carefully monitored. 200 mg prednisolone may be needed initially. The usefulness of methotrexate rests in the fact that the dosage of prednisolone can be greatly reduced, when the two are used in combination, the aim being the ultimate withdrawal of steroids.

The patient must be kept in bed for the preliminary study. Secondary infection must be avoided.

Locally, the lesions can be treated with potassium permanganate or eusol dressings, whilst in generalized cases, potassium permanganate baths are useful.

PROGNOSIS

This depends on the response to treatment, yet nearly 50 per cent of patients die within 6 months to 10 years of the onset.

Pemphigoid

Bullous pemphigoid

This fairly uncommon disorder is characterized by large, tense bullae (Fig. 42), occurring in elderly people. The onset is sudden. The

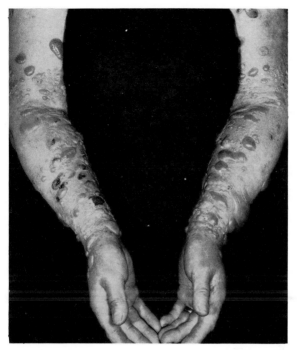

FIG. 42. Pemphigoid (Institute of Dermatology, University of London).

bullae are tough and do not break easily, containing clear, straw-coloured fluid. The arms and thighs are always involved, and any other area less often. Oral lesions, and sometimes ocular ones, are a feature of the disease, occurring in about 20 per cent of cases.

The cause is unknown, but like pemphigus it may be an immuno-suppressive disease. It is relatively benign. The lesions are sub-epidermal which differentiates it histologically from pemphigus, and therefore acantholysis is absent.

Methotrexate and/or steroids are invariably effective.

TABLE 2

Differential diagnosis of bullous eruptions

	Dermatitis Herpetiformis	Pemphigus	Pemphigoid
Age	Any	Usually 40–60	Over 60
Sex	Both	Both	Both
Eruption	Vesicles, and bullae	Bullae	Bullae
Site	Lumbo-sacral, buttocks, post. axillary folds common. Lesions are grouped	Face, neck, trunk, limbs. No grouping	Thighs, arms, trunk
Mucous membranes	Oral mucosa sometimes affected	Commonly affected	Affected in about 20 per cent of cases
Itching	Always present, and may be severe	Rare	Rare
Pathology	Subepidermal bullae No acantholysis	Intra-epidermal bullae Acantholysis present	Both types No acantholysis
Eosinophilia	10–40 per cent	Usual, but low	Unusual
Course	Chronic	Chronic	Chronic
Treatment	Dapsone	Steroids Methotrexate	Steroids methotrexate
Prognosis	Disease lasts 5–20 years	Fairly good with modern therapy	Quite good

TABLE 3

Indirect immunofluorescence (IIF) findings

	Dermatitis Herpetiformis	Pemphigus	Pemphigoid
Type of IF	None	In intra-cellular zone	In basement membrane zone
Type of Ig	None	IgG	IgG
Complement fixing		Yes	Yes

CHAPTER 13

Diseases due to Parasites

Scabies: Pediculosis: Fleas: Bed Bugs:
Bees: Wasps: Ants: Cheyletiella

Scabies

This is a contagious disease caused by infestation with *Sarcoptes scabiei* (*Acarus scabiei*, Fig. 43), characterized by intra-epidermal burrows and follicular papules, and severe itching which is worse at night.

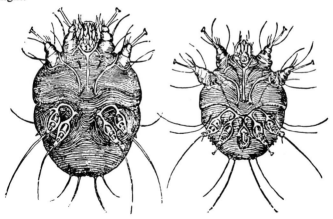

Fig. 43. *Acarus scabiei*, ventral surface. The female is the larger.

PARASITOLOGY

The female acarus is pearly grey, with 4 pairs of legs, is oval in shape and can be seen quite easily on the end of a pin, or on a glass slide. The male is seldom seen, as copulation proves to be fatal.

The pregnant acarus burrows into the horny layer of the skin into which she lays her eggs. The burrow is $\frac{1}{4}$ to $\frac{1}{2}$ an inch in length, with a roof that appears as a whitish zig-zag line, punctuated by one or more black specks which are caused by dirt or faeces in the burrow. The acarus may be found at the farthest end of the burrow by inserting a needle and gently breaking the roof at that point, followed by judicious probing which will cause the acarus to hang on the end of the needle.

The eggs hatch in 3–4 days, and six-legged larvae leave the burrow to find shelter in hair-follicles. They then slough their skin, twice, becoming eight-legged, and within 14–17 days adult females on impregnation initiate the cycle again.

Eggs	→	3–4 days later larvae	→	2 weeks later after moultings adult acari

10–25 eggs may be laid during the life of a female.

Other varieties of scabies are horse, dog and cat scabies which may attack people in contact with them. One per cent of dogs in the U.K. are carriers.

Transmission
of the disease is by close and prolonged contact. It is usually contracted in bed from an infested companion or occasionally spread indirectly by bedding.

CLINICAL FEATURES
Remarkably severe itching occurs predominantly at night in bed, for that is the time when the person is warm and the mite prefers to promenade.

The onset is gradual. Lesions apart from burrows and papules also consist of pustules, excoriations, and crusted lesions. Sites of the burrows are the ulnar borders of the wrists, the palms, fingers, the anterior axillary folds, areolae of the nipples, lower abdomen, buttocks and penis (Fig. 44). Other lesions may occur anywhere. The skin above the neck-line is rarely, if ever, affected because the acarus avoids the cold as much as possible.

The extension of scabies may be promoted and/or masked by the use of potent topical steroids.

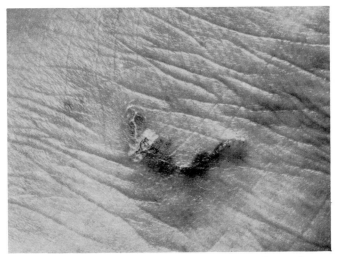

Fig. 44. Scabies: a typical burrow on the palm, with haemorrhage due to scratching. In the intact area on the right a black speck identifies the situation of the acarus (Institute of Dermatology, University of London).

DIAGNOSIS

When lesions are minimal, scabies must often be consciously considered, and careful examination will reveal burrows. The social status of the person must never be taken into account for, like the flea, the acarus is not class-conscious. In well-developed cases, nocturnal itching and burrows are well established.

TREATMENT

Benzyl benzoate application B.P., containing 25 per cent benzyl benzoate, a cream containing 1 per cent gamma benzene hexachloride (Lorexane), or monosulfiram (Tetmosol) 25 per cent in an alcoholic base, diluted with 4 parts of water, is applied from the neck down following a hot bath, during which burrows are gently rubbed open with a soft brush. About 50 ml of the chosen remedy are required.

Two days later a bath may be taken followed by a change of bed linen and underclothing, the soiled articles being dealt with by ordinary laundering, and not by disinfestation.

Residual itching following this treatment should be dealt with by calamine lotion, and not more scabiecides. Treatment may fail for various reasons in 5 per cent of cases, and may be repeated 2–3 weeks after the first course. Finally, all contacts should be treated.

Pediculosis

This means infestation by lice. There are 3 types (Fig. 45):

1. *Pediculus capitis*—head louse.
2. *Pediculus corporis*—body louse.
3. *Phthirus pubis*—crab louse.

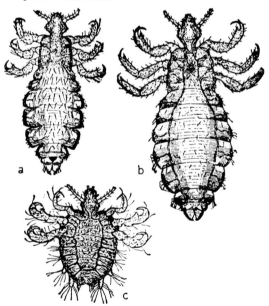

FIG. 45. Pediculi: dorsal surfaces of females. (a) *P. capitis*, (b) *P. corporis*, (c) *P. pubis*.

PARASITOLOGY

Lice are oval and grey, about 2–4 mm long, wingless, and have 6 legs.
Pubic lice are the smallest, and body lice are the largest. The female,
whose life-span is 1 month, lays several hundred eggs, called nits,
each one being glued on to a hair. A larva is hatched out in 6–10 days,
and becomes a fully grown louse in 1 or 2 weeks.

Nit   →   In 6–10 days   →   1–2 weeks later
                            larva   after 3 moultings
                                                              louse

They live on blood, which they suck from the skin, and only attack
live humans. Each louse rarely leaves its own territory, except in
severe infestations.

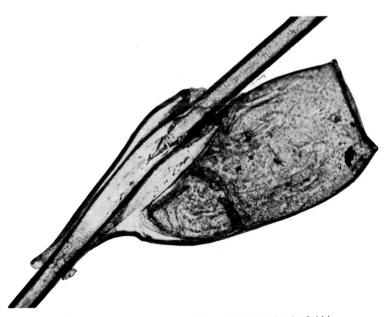

FIG. 46. Nit or ovum glued to a hair by a cylindrical sheath of chitin.

Pediculosis Capitis

This is found chiefly in women and girls, especially at the back and sides of the scalp. As a result of scratching, impetigo occurs, and enlargement of the occipital glands. The eyelashes may also be involved. The translucent nits can be seen glued to the hair (Fig. 46), and are difficult to remove. A watchful eye may see a louse moving on the scalp.

The diagnosis must be firmly made before informing the patient. Infestation is considered by some to be a terrible disgrace, and if the patient is wrongly informed the physician's reputation will suffer disproportionately.

TREATMENT

Dicophane application B.P.C., 2 per cent, or 0·2 per cent gamma benzene hexachloride application B.P.C., is rubbed into the hair once. Both remain to some extent even after washing, and lice are killed by traces of it. When these remedies are not available, benzyl benzoate application, B.P., may be used. The hair need not be cut. Contacts must also be treated.

In cases of lice and nits resistant to gammexane, malathion lotion 0·5% in spirit is effective, although cases of lice resistant to this have also been recorded.

Lindane powder may be applied to the backs of chairs, etc., where heads may have rested.

Pediculosis Corporis

This louse lives in clothes, and only leaves them to have a meal off the skin. The eggs are laid in the underclothing. Scratch marks are the only lesion of this infestation. Body lice are the cause of typhus, trench fever, and relapsing fever.

TREATMENT

is by giving the patient a hot bath, and following this with the application of dicophane dusting powder, not forgetting the underclothes.

Pediculosis Pubis

This may be contracted during sexual intercourse, or from bedding.

It is commonly found in the pubic area, but also in the axillae, and on the eyelashes and chest. Itching may be severe, and the louse should be looked for in cases of pruritus ani and vulvae (Fig. 47).

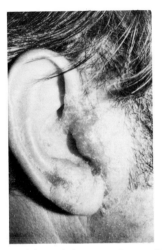

FIG. 47. Impetiginous lesions secondary to *P. capitis.*

TREATMENT

is the same as for *P. capitis.*

Fleas

They are brown, wingless, flat insects, with 3 pairs of legs, and have the power to jump huge distances in relation to their size. Their bite (to which many people are relatively immune) produces a haemorrhagic spot surrounded by an itchy wheal. They may also be the cause of papular urticaria.

TREATMENT

is by spraying carpets, cracks in floors, domestic animals and their baskets with dicophane dusting powder. To catch a flea is an art; a piece of moist soap and a white surface like a bath or a sheet are required for it to jump on, as it is inclined to be attracted to such a colour. A steroid lotion is a good anti-pruritic.

Bedbug

It is yellowish-brown, oval, with 3 pairs of legs, and is twice as big as a louse. It is said by specialists to have a nasty smell. It lives in cracks in furniture, and can do so without food for a year. They may be the cause of papular urticaria.

Bites are grouped in twos or threes, especially round the ankles and buttocks.

Crevices in furniture should be sprayed with dicophane dusting powder.

Bees, Wasps, Ants

Chronic urticaria can result from the sting of these insects, as well as generalized formication and granulomata.

Bee poison is acid and ammonia or sodium bicarbonate should be applied, after extraction of the sting.

Wasp poison is alkaline, or neutral, and should be treated with lemon juice or vinegar.

Insect bites occasionally produce bullous lesions.

Antihistamines by mouth are useful for reducing pruritus and oedema. Bee-keepers should store a tube of adrenaline, which can be self-administered, for severe reactions.

Cheyletiella

C. parasitovorax and *C. yasguri* have recently been found more often in the U.K., being isolated from dogs, cats, and rabbits. It is an acarine-like parasite. Human lesions occur in crops, in small groups, or are scattered. They start as itchy, red macules, becoming vesiculo-pustular and then crusted.

Treatment of infested animals alone may suffice, but in chronic cases, furniture and coverings may also need attention.

CHAPTER 14

Disturbances of Pigmentation

Freckles: Chloasma: Albinism: Vitiligo

Pigment may be increased in the skin, or, in some conditions, diminished; however, hyper-pigmentation is more common than hypo-pigmentation. There are a great many conditions which come into both categories, and only the common ones will be dealt with here.

The principal causes for hyper-pigmentation are:

(1) Increase of melanin, which may be local or general, and more rarely:
(2) Deposits of foreign pigments.
(3) Deposits of heavy metals, e.g. arsenic.
(4) Deposits of haemoglobin derivatives, as in haemosiderosis.

The common conditions characterized by hyper-pigmentation are:

Local	General
Freckles	Cushing's syndrome
Pigmented naevi	Addison's disease
Chloasma	Haemochromatosis
	Scleroderma

Freckles

These are caused by sunlight. They are common in blonde individuals and tend to fade in winter. They may be removed with the application of carbon-dioxide snow (30–40 secs). Sunscreening agents are usually ineffective.

Chloasma

Melasma

This describes brownish patches on the face of the pregnant woman, due to the melanocyte-stimulating hormone of the pituitary gland. They disappear at the end of pregnancy. Occasionally it appears on non-pregnant women, and sometimes oral contraceptives induce it.

Pigmented naevi

These are dealt with in chapter 20.

Common conditions characterized by hypo-pigmentation are:

Local	*General*
Vitiligo	Vitiligo
	Albinism

Albinism

This is a congenital absence of melanin involving the hair, eyes, and skin.

It is more common in males, and there is usually a familial or hereditary history. It is seen in all races.

The skin is a delicate pink, the hair a silky white, the eyes are pink, and the person's sensitivity to light is noticeable: he blinks his eyelids and stands with cast-down eyes. Keratoses and epitheliomata are liable to occur later in life, as a reaction to the activity of the sun.

No treatment is effective, but the skin and eyes must be shaded from sunlight. Life in temperate zones is preferable to that in tropical ones.

Vitiligo or Leucoderma

A condition in which pigment disappears from the skin in patches, so that they become white (Fig. 48).

CAUSE

This is unknown, although recent findings suggest auto-immune factors. Dark people are commonly affected in both sexes and at any age; however, 50 per cent of cases develop between infancy and the age of 20, quite often in infancy. A familial history is often revealed.

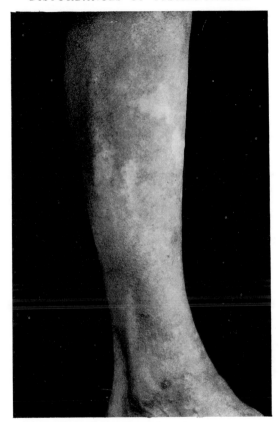

FIG. 48. Vitiligo (leucoderma) of the leg.

CLINICAL FEATURES

The onset is sudden. The patches assume various sizes and shapes and are commonest on the face and neck, hands and wrists, abdomen and thighs. Hair may also become white. All these patches are very sensitive to sunlight.

Vitiligo may be associated with certain systemic disorders; notably, pernicious anaemia, hyperthyroidism, diabetes and perhaps with neoplasms in the case of elderly patients. Other skin disorders such as alopecia areata, psoriasis or eczema, may co-exist.

COURSE

The condition can remain static for months or years, and only occasionally clears spontaneously.

DIAGNOSIS

In widespread cases it is easy to confuse the vitiliginous condition, with one of hyper-pigmentation. It may seem that the individual has a white skin peppered with dark patches which, in contrast with the white, are very dark indeed. The true state of affairs can be made clear by examining the edge of the white areas. If it is convex, the condition is one of vitiligo. If in doubt, examine for the superficial scales of pityriasis versicolor (p. 142).

TREATMENT

There is none which is very satisfactory.

8-Methoxypsoralen (Methoxsalen) taken orally produces re-pigmentation in some cases of vitiligo, and so far there have not been any reports of toxic effects.

For those under 12 years of age, 10 mg twice weekly is given, and for those over 12, 20–40 mg daily. Two hours after taking the tablet, the affected areas are exposed to ultra-violet radiation, that from natural sunlight, administered for a specified period, being the more effective, the aim being gradually to reach a point at which a perceptible erythema can be maintained in them. Patients between the ages of 3 and 60 have been treated for periods varying from 3 months to 3 years.

Betamethasone valerate 0·1 per cent (Betnovate) in a cream base, or in isopropyl alcohol 50 per cent of clobetasol propionate (Dermovate) cream applied twice daily without exposure to ultra-violet light may be even more effective, but the usual dangers must be considered as with all potent steroids (p. 30).

CHAPTER 15

Diseases due to Metabolic or Hormonal Disorders

Xanthomata: Vitamin Deficiencies: Acromegaly:
Cushing's Syndrome: Myxoedema: Diabetes Mellitus:
Addison's Disease: Pregnancy

In these conditions, the skin lesions play a very minor role as regards the health of the patient, but their recognition, in some cases, is a major clue to the underlying diagnosis. The condition most noticeably absent from this chapter is acne vulgaris, which is dealt with on page 202.

METABOLIC DISORDERS

Xanthomata

These are yellowish or pinkish—yellowish papules, or nodules (Plate 27), containing cholesterol fat. There are two varieties.

(1) Xanthoma planum
in which yellow papules or plaques form in the skin of the eyelids, generally of middle-aged women. The blood cholesterol is raised in over two-thirds of all cases.

TREATMENT
consists of excision, or the very careful application of tri-chlor-acetic acid by an experienced person, resulting in a scab, which disintegrates within 2 or 3 weeks. In many cases, no treatment is required.

(2) Xanthoma tuberosum
which, as might be gathered, consists of larger, nodular lesions. They appear on the extensor surfaces. The mucous membranes may also

be involved. The blood cholesterol is always raised. Large nodules
can be excised.

Vitamin Deficiencies

Vitamin A (Carotene)
This is characterized by dryness and roughness of the skin, usually
of the fronts of the thighs and the back of the forearms. The hands
and feet usually remain unaffected.

Vitamin D (dihydroxycholecalciferol)
This causes no skin lesions.

Vitamin E (toferol)
There is no concrete evidence that this is responsible for skin lesions.

Vitamin B$_1$ (Nicotinamide)
This causes no skin lesions, unless combined with vitamin B$_2$
deficiency, when pellagra ensues.

Pellagra
This is characterized by symmetrical redness and scaliness of areas
exposed to light, namely, the wrists, ankles, face and neck. Weeks
or months later, peeling occurs and is followed by pigmentation.

The pellagrinous nose—redness and scaling of the bridge—is
characteristic.

Pellagra is recognized by the 3 D's of dermatitis, diarrhoea and
dementia.

Other signs of this deficiency are a sore tongue, inflamed lips,
anorexia, weight loss and insomnia.

TREATMENT
is by giving nicotinamide 500 mg daily by mouth, and 50 mg daily
intra-muscularly, apart from bed-rest, and a diet rich in the vitamin
B complex.

Vitamin B$_2$ (Riboflavin)
Skin lesions are characterized by redness and fissuring of the angles
of the mouth (angular cheilitis). In severe cases, the tongue becomes
magenta coloured.

HORMONAL DISORDERS

Acromegaly

There may be many skin changes, and these include thickening and furrowing of the skin of the face, with seborrhoea and hirsuties. The nose becomes broad, and the ears, lower lip and tongue markedly thicker. The nails become broad, thickened, and sometimes spoon-shaped.

Cushing's syndrome

Many notable skin changes may accompany this disorder, which is due to a basophil adenoma of the pituitary, or to hyperplasia or a tumour of the adrenal cortex.

The skin may be hirsute, dusky and plethoric, accompanied by purpura and ecchymoses, and remarkable striae distensae.

All these signs may arise too as a result of steroid administration.

Myxoedema

Hypothyroidism

In this condition, the skin, hair and nails are affected. The skin is dry, uncomfortably rough, swollen and waxy, this colour being due to myxoedema. Although the skin is swollen, there is no pitting oedema. The hair of the scalp is dry and thin, and has none of its normal lustre. Examination of the hair of the eyebrows will reveal a definite loss of their outer two-thirds, and pubic and axillary hair will be absent or very sparse. The nails are brittle and ridged.

A *localized* form of the above condition may occur on the fronts of the legs, and is called pre-tibial myxoedema. It may or may not be associated with thyroid insufficiency.

Diabetes Mellitus

This condition may be accompanied by boils or carbuncles, pruritus, leg ulcers, or xanthomata.

Boils and pruritus are common conditions; however, in a busy clinic where all urines cannot be tested, urine examination should never be left out when there is a history of boils or pruritus even though the test has been made elsewhere! The number of cases in which glycosuria is present is very small, so that sometimes one despairs of finding sugar in the urine. But when one is least expecting it, a case will arise, rewarding perseverance.

Addison's Disease

The pigmentation in this disease is light to dark brown, and affects exposed surfaces, except the palms and creases.

Pregnancy and skin lesions

The incidence of eruptions during pregnancy is less than 1 per cent. They usually appear after the fifth month, and disappear early in the post-natal period. Various erythematous eruptions may occur, and pruritus or urticaria.

Frontal alopecia occurs occasionally. During pregnancy conversion from ana- to telogen is slowed (see p. 5); and in the post-partum period conversion is accelerated, so that 2–4 months after parturition frontal alopecia may appear. Reassurance that the hair loss will cease in 2–5 months, and that complete regrowth will occur, is necessary.

CHAPTER 16

Diseases due to Vascular Disorders

Varicose Dermatitis: Purpuras

The commonest skin disorders under this heading are those due to stasis in the vessels, and comprise such conditions as varicose dermatitis, thrombo-phlebitis of the leg, and congestive cardiac failure with a rise in venous back-pressure. Purpuric eruptions also come under this heading.

Varicose Dermatitis and Ulcer

The skin conditions produced by varicose veins are dermatitis and ulceration and they are, unfortunately, very common in the practice of skin diseases.

The cause of the eruption is nearly always a former thrombo-phlebitis, which in a great many cases the patient cannot recall, either because it occurred a few years before the appearance of the skin lesions, or because the discomfort was so minimal that it passed unnoticed. Middle-aged women outnumber men by about 4 to 1. Overweight and heredity may play minor roles in their causation.

CLINICAL FEATURES

The onset is insidious with moderate oedema of the inner aspects of the ankles. This tends to wax and wane, depending on the amount of standing the patient has to do. (Walking is far less harmful as it constantly maintains a venous flow.) Poorly-defined areas of redness then develop, and gradually dry or moist scaly lesions appear. These become itchy, and owing to scratching or minor trauma, an ulcer develops. The ulcers have soft irregular edges, become infected, and give off a most offensive smell. They involve areas from the size of a two-pence piece to that of a five-pound note or larger (Fig. 49), and can be very painful. Both legs may be affected.

As the disease progresses, there is always a danger of eczematization of the skin, and an eczematous eruption occurring at first around the ulcer may then spread widely over the body.

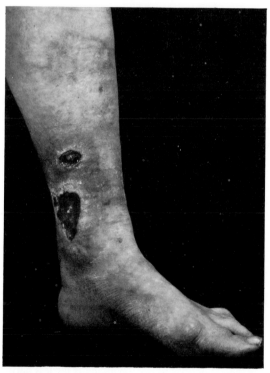

FIG. 49. Varicose ulcers: 10 years' recurrent ulceration (Skin Department, London Hospital).

DIAGNOSIS

When dermatitis is present, localized neurodermatitis must be excluded. This is never associated with oedema of the ankles, and is extremely itchy.

When an ulcer develops, hypertension and arteriosclerosis must be considered, but here the ulcers are small and punched out, and usually extremely painful. Malignancy, gummata and erythema induratum are possibilities in some cases, but then there is no evidence of venous stasis. Less common causes of leg ulcers are, for example, chilblains, ulcerative colitis, and rheumatoid arthritis.

TREATMENT

For thrombophlebitis
firm bandaging, and anti-coagulants if necessary.

For dermatitis
a bland ointment or cream containing calamine or a steroid cream are often effective. Nothing must be applied which could possibly cause sensitivity of the skin, which is, in this condition, in a very delicate state. Antibiotic ointments should only be given after careful thought. If the rash is very severe, a short term of bed-rest may be necessary. When the rash has cleared, supportive treatment for the leg in the form of elastic stockings or bandages must be instituted indefinitely. A surgeon's opinion should be sought concerning the advisability of operative treatment.

For ulcers
the aim is to avoid anything encouraging venous stasis, and the accumulation of oedema, and to improve the blood supply.

Bed-rest should be avoided unless there is gross infection of the ulcer and surrounding oedema. Even then, it should only be employed to bring the condition initially under control. Then the foot of the bed should be raised, and a cradle introduced under the bed-clothes to take their weight off the leg. Long periods of bed-rest are definitely harmful.

Ambulant treatment is best for ulcers, and this is made possible by bandaging. The following methods are effective:

1. Daily applications of eusol on gauze, followed by an elastic bandage from knee to foot. It is essential that the patient is shown the correct way to apply it, and a nursing sister is the best person to do this.

2. Occlusive paste medicated bandages. A zinc or calamine bandage impregnated with iodochlorhydroxyquinoline (Quina-band) is applied to the leg from the knee to the foot, and changed at weekly intervals.

3. Crepe bandaging. A polyurethane foam pad is placed over the ulcer and kept in position by a length of tubular gauze. Compression is then obtained with a cotton crepe or poroplast bandage. This outer bandage may be removed at night-time, and reapplied each morning.

Finally, physiotherapy in the form of massage and exercises is very helpful in reducing oedema and induration.

PROGNOSIS

The future health of the leg depends on the patient's recognition of the importance of avoiding trauma of any kind, of avoiding long periods of standing, and the wearing of a supportive elastic bandage when the slightest oedema is present.

Purpura

This term is used to describe the appearance of purple-red spots in the skin or mucous membranes, due to haemorrhage from capillaries. It is not a disease in itself, but a sign of an underlying condition. The causes are innumerable, and sometimes difficult to discover.

The causes may be grouped under two headings: (A) Capillary wall defects; (B) Blood defects.

(A) CAPILLARY WALL DEFECTS

This may be a generalized or a localized condition. If the former, the tourniquet test will be positive. If the latter, it will be negative. In both cases, the platelet count should be normal, i.e., 200,000–500,000.

The following are common causes of this variety of purpura:

1. Simple purpura.
2. Senile purpura.
3. Venous-stasis purpura.
4. Drugs; also responsible for purpura associated with blood defects.
5. Avitaminosis; e.g. scurvy.
6. Systemic diseases; also responsible for purpura associated with blood defects.
7. Henoch-Schoenlein syndrome (allergic purpura).

1. SIMPLE PURPURA

This mild form of purpura is found in association with sensitivity to certain bacterial infections, especially streptococcal. Thus, it is seen in rheumatic fever, scarlet fever, etc., and slight constitutional symptoms may or may not be present.

2. SENILE PURPURA

This is similar to the childhood variety, but is due to degeneration of the tissue supporting the capillaries.

3. VENOUS STASIS PURPURA

This variety occurs around the ankles and lower parts of the legs due to varicose veins, and also in fat men in the absence of varicose veins. It is accompanied by progressive pigmentation and the deposition of haemosiderin, so that a cayenne-pepper appearance develops.

4. DRUGS

Many drugs can produce a purpuric reaction. Among a few commonly responsible, the following should be noted: sulphonamides, chloramphenicol, phenylbutazone, indomethacin, tolbutamide, methotrexate.

5. SCURVY

The pathognomic sign is the appearance of swollen and spongy gums in the region of the papillae, between the teeth. Purpura is often found on the thighs, just above the knees. The haemorrhages are peri-follicular.

6. SYSTEMIC DISEASES

Again only a few will be named. These are: subacute bacterial endocarditis, scarlet fever, measles, meningitis, typhoid fever, diabetes, hypertension and chronic nephritis.

7. HENOCH-SCHOENLEIN SYNDROME (Allergic purpura)

This type occurs in children and adolescents, and is characterized by a special sequence of lesions, as well as gastrointestinal and arthritic symptoms.

CLINICAL FEATURES

These are commonly preceded by an upper respiratory infection occurring one or two weeks before other signs.

The earliest lesion is a dark red purpuric papule, which becomes successively vesicular or bullous and then ulcerates. Sites commonly affected are the buttocks and the extensor aspects of the limbs, the distribution being symmetrical.

Peri-articular effusions may cause painful swellings of the joints. Mild fever is normal.

The gastrointestinal symptoms are in the form of epigastric pain, and sometimes haematemesis and melaena, often imitating appendicitis or intussusception.

TREATMENT

Symptomatic and bed-rest, which clears up the attack in a week or two. In severe cases, steroids have been used with success.

(B) BLOOD DEFECTS

The common defect is thrombocytopenia. Defects in clotting, and plasma protein abnormalities are rare.

When purpura is present, a platelet count and other relevant clotting investigations should always be made.

The common conditions producing thrombocytopenic purpura are as follows:

1. Idiopathic, or primary thrombocytopenic purpura.

2. Drug purpura; also a cause of the non-thrombocytopenic variety.

3. Systemic diseases: also responsible for the non-thrombocytopenic variety.

1. IDIOPATHIC THROMBOCYTOPENIC PURPURA

There are two forms: (i) acute, and self-limiting, occurring in children, frequently following a viral infection; (ii) chronic, being associated with splenomegaly, and found in young adults. In some instances these may be due to an antigen–antibody reaction.

For the chronic form, the following treatments should be considered: steroid therapy, and splenectomy.

2. DRUG PURPURA

See under purpura due to capillary defects.

3. SYSTEMIC DISEASES

Here other more grave conditions should be considered, such as leukaemia, acute or chronic, aplastic anaemia, splenic disorders such as Kala-azar or malaria, systemic lupus erythematosus, or generalized carcinomatosis.

TREATMENT

The treatment of all purpuric eruptions depends on the cause, and when the condition is systemic a general physician should be consulted.

CHAPTER 17

Systemic Diseases of Unknown Cause

Lupus Erythematosus: Sarcoidosis: Scleroderma:
Dermatomyositis: Reiter's Disease

LUPUS ERYTHEMATOSUS

This condition appears in two distinct forms:

1. Localized, or chronic.
2. Systemic, or acute.

Chronic

The *chronic type* is characterized by inflammatory, scaly, round papular lesions, usually distributed symmetrically on the face (Plates 28, 29). It commonly remains localized to the skin, but may occasionally become systemic and fatal.

CAUSE

This is unknown precisely, although the condition appears to be one of the connective tissue, and an auto-immunological disorder, anti-nuclear factor being found in about 20 per cent of cases.

PREDISPOSING FACTORS ARE

Sex: women are more affected than men, in a ratio of 9:3.

PATHOLOGY

The classical changes in this disease are: (1) hyperkeratosis, which notably plugs the follicles (Fig. 50), and which is also a diagnostic clinical sign; (2) alternating acanthosis and atrophy of the prickle-cell layer; (3) liquefaction degeneration of the basal layer, so that this layer is separated by a cleft from the dermis; (4) a peri-vascular lymphocytic infiltrate seen chiefly around the appendages of the dermis. Other less typical changes may or may not be present.

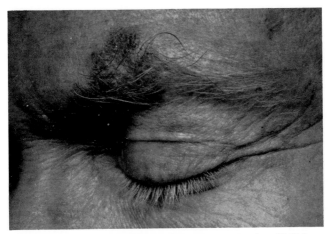

Fig. 50. Chronic lupus erythematosus showing the plugging of follicles by scales, so-called follicular hyperkeratosis.

CLINICAL FEATURES

The onset is insidious. The lesions are papular, usually about pea-size, and enlarging very slowly to 30 mm diameter or larger. They are normally round or oval, and very close examination of the scaly surface will reveal that the scales in many areas appear as dots; these dots indicate where the follicle has been plugged by a scale, and when scales are removed and the undersurface is inspected they clearly appear as tiny spicules projecting from the scaly mass. No other scaly condition produces this phenomenon.

Sites commonly affected are the face, particularly the cheeks and nose (the so-called butterfly area of the face, the cheeks being the imaginary wings of the butterfly, Fig. 51), the ears and the scalp. The mucous membranes of the lips and mouth may be attacked and show sharply defined, slightly raised whitish patches, with red borders. When the lips themselves are involved, they are covered with very closely bound scales.

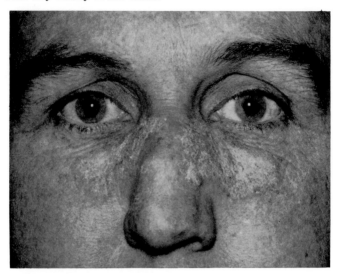

Fig. 51. Discoid lupus erythematosus: involvement of the so-called butterfly area of the face (Department of Dermatology, Addenbrooke's Hospital).

Investigations

Blood count, urine, and sedimentation rate should be checked, as well as an L.E. cell preparation; the ESR is raised in 25 per cent of cases, and L.E. cells are found in about 10 per cent.

COURSE

The lesions heal with flat and slightly depressed scars. Relapses are common, and may continue for many years. But above all, a watchful eye must be kept on all active cases of chronic lupus erythematosus. A small percentage of them may develop into the dreaded systemic type, described below. This is refuted by some authors, who consider the acute and chronic types to be different entities. There is no unanimity about this.

DIAGNOSIS

This is made by the appearance of scaly discoid lesions (Fig. 52), with the unique plugging of the follicles. The condition must be distinguished from (1) *lupus vulgaris*, which tends to ulcerate the skin, and in which there is no follicular plugging; (2) *eczema*, which is itchy,

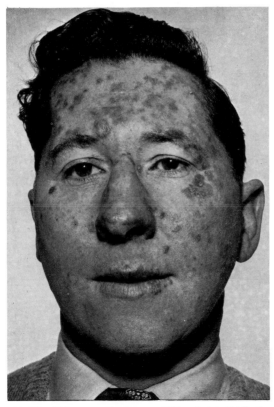

Fig. 52. Discoid lupus erythematosus. Diffuse facial distribution of lesions (Dr E. Waddington).

and whose evolution is more rapid; (3) *psoriasis*, which has loosely adherent silvery scales, usually with evidence of the condition elsewhere; (4) *seborrhoeic dermatitis*, which shows greasy loose scales; (5) when appearing on the hands, *chilblains* must be excluded.

TREATMENT

Patients must avoid sunlight, and when out-of-doors wear wide-brimmed hats. Antibiotics must be avoided, as they may disseminate the disease.

The following treatments may be used:

Steroids applied as creams or ointments.
Steroids by injection into the lesion.
Steroids by mouth.
Chloroquine sulphate (Nivaquine) or
Hydroxy-chloroquine (Plaquenil) tablets.

Betamethasone valerate (Betnovate) and fluocinolone acetonide (Synalar) creams rubbed in twice daily suppress most lesions. For deeply infiltrated lesions, intralesional injections of triamcinolone can be given. Chloroquine (Nivaquine) 200 mg tablets 2 or 3 times a day may be given as a last resort, providing no side-effects occur (see p. 35), and even so, used only during spring and summer months under constant supervision.

Systemic

The *acute disseminated type* of lupus erythematosus is a progressive and grave disease. It affects every organ in the body, and in only half the cases is there skin involvement.

It is uncommon, affecting about 4/100,000 of the British population; 90 per cent of cases occur in females, usually between the ages of 20 and 40 years.

CAUSE

This is unknown, although there is substantial evidence that it is due to an allergic auto-immune reaction, as shown by the production of auto-antibodies, cf. the L.E. phenomenon, Coombs' test, and A.N.F. test.

The patient stricken with systemic L.E. is particularly vulnerable to many reactions which may act as a trigger mechanism. The effect of sunlight on a skin lesion may result in the development of an acute exacerbation. Drug reactions, among others, to sulphonamides and penicillin may also produce the same effect.

Another pointer to the cause may lie in the fact that connective tissue is the target area, degenerative changes being found in the mesenchymal tissues of all organs attacked.

The L.E. Phenomenon

This phenomenon is seen in blood smears, as a result of a special examination of the patient's plasma or serum, when mixed with normal heparinized marrow, or whole blood. The L.E. cell may then be seen. It is a leucocyte, engulfing a round, smoky, basophilic mass of nucleoprotein.

The L.E. phenomenon is always positive at some time in systemic L.E. and in chronic L.E. in about 10 per cent of cases. It is now largely superseded by the A.N.F. test.

PATHOLOGY

Skin changes when present are relatively similar to those of the chronic variety.

Visceral changes commonly found are: (1) verrucous endocarditis (Libman-Sacks syndrome); (2) renal lesions producing a nephrotic syndrome; (3) pleurisy or pericarditis. A vasculitis of the C.N.S. may also occur, and the skeletal muscles may be affected.

CLINICAL FEATURES

Languor, weakness, anorexia, loss of weight, low-grade pyrexia, chest pains, vague joint symptoms.

Skin lesions are present in only 50 per cent of cases (Plate 30). Other clinical signs are legion, as any organ may be attacked.

Laboratory investigations will reveal albuminuria, haematuria, leucopenia, anaemia, thrombocytopenia, a very high sedimentation rate, and hypergammaglobulinaemia.

DIAGNOSIS

If classical skin lesions are present it is straightforward. If not, it is based on the laboratory findings and clinical signs. Rheumatic fever and bacterial endocarditis must be excluded.

TREATMENT

Sunlight and offensive drugs must be avoided.

Bed-rest, good nursing and feeding are essential. Steroids must be given, and at first in high doses; e.g. prednisolone 80–100 mg daily. Reduction of the dose must be gentle and slow. Anti-malarials, e.g. chloroquine, also have a place in treatment (see p. 34).

This is but an outline of the treatment of one of the most challenging diseases in medicine.

PROGNOSIS

This is always grave, and depends on many factors such as the extent of the disease and its response to steroids.

Sarcoidosis

This is a chronic systemic disease, which produces papules, nodules or plaques in the skin in about one-third of the cases.

The pathological reaction is a reticulo-endothelial one, and the disease prefers organs containing a large amount of reticulo-endothelial tissue.

The term sarcoid is derived from the Greek word *sarx*, meaning flesh. Sarcoid is a misleading term, as it suggests a relationship to sarcoma erroneously. Like many other misnomers in medical terminology, it is too deeply embedded to be eradicated.

The condition is commonest in females, and between the ages of 20 and 40.

CAUSE

This is unknown. The disorder bears a faint resemblance to tuberculosis, clinically, but the relationship to it is very doubtful. A viral cause has been cited but never proved.

PATHOLOGY

The most characteristic feature is the presence of well-defined clumps, resembling nests, of epithelioid cells. Once seen, they are unmistakable. Their position in the skin varies according to the type of skin lesion present. This epithelioid infiltration is the same whether it involves the lungs, bones, viscera or skin. Caseation is rare, giant cells are occasionally present, and tubercle bacilli never.

CLINICAL FEATURES

Skin changes occur in nearly 50 per cent of cases of sarcoidosis. The commonest cutaneous indication is erythema nodosum (see p. 85). But specific skin changes also occur.

The onset is gradual. The lesions are papules, nodules or plaques. They may be any shape, and are quite well defined (Plate 31). They are reddish-brown, and vary in number from one to a hundred or more. The surface of the skin is usually unchanged, and the granulomatous infiltrate can be sensed by palpation. This varies in degree, depending on whether the infiltrate is dermal or subcutaneous. The commonest sites are the face, neck, and back of the arms.

In patients with active sarcoidosis, an intra-epidermal injection of a ground-up suspension of sarcoid tissue from an active source evokes a papular reaction, appearing 7–10 days later, and persisting, often for several months. The resultant nodule is excised, and examined histologically. This is the Kveim test.

COURSE

The lesions usually fade without leaving a mark, after months or years, although occasionally atrophy and scarring occur.

Other signs

which may occur are very varied, and consist of (1) lymphadeno-pathy, in 80 per cent of cases, usually involving the cervical, axillary, or inguinal groups; (2) lung changes in 75 per cent of cases; (3) bone involvement, presenting as a non-ulcerative dactylitis of the fingers and toes; and (4) granular uveitis, which may lead to blindness.

DIAGNOSIS

This is made by the Kveim test.

The histology provides further confirmation; approaching 100 per cent of lymph nodes show identifiable granulomatous change even without obvious lymphadenopathy.

Diascopy may be helpful where the lesion shows a brownish colour similar to lupus vulgaris. The blood can show an increase in protein, particularly hypergammaglobulinaemia.

TREATMENT

When the condition is localized to the skin, none is indicated, as the lesions ultimately resolve without it, but should it be apparent that the disease is systemic, steroids must be given.

PROGNOSIS
Cutaneous lesions tend to recur.

SCLERODERMA

This is a disorder characterized by induration of the skin. It exists in two forms: (1) localized; (2) systemic. The cause is unknown.

PATHOLOGY
The chief changes are fibrosis and sclerosis of the collagen fibres, and sclerotic and obliterative changes in the vessels. In later stages, there is universal atrophy of the appendages in the dermis, and elastic tissue becomes fragmented.

When the condition is generalized, grosser changes occur, such as sclerosis and atrophy of the skeletal muscle bundles. The oesophageal, intestinal and cardiac musculature is also often involved, and is clearly reflected in the clinical signs.

Localized Scleroderma

This is also known as morphoea, and consists of localized patches of hardened white atrophic skin.

CLINICAL FEATURES
The onset is gradual. The lesion may be pea to palm size, varying in its rate of growth. The shape may be oval, round or linear, and in recent lesions is edged with a definite pale violet hem. Later it disappears. The surface is hard and smooth, and the lesion is difficult to lift. There may be one or several lesions, and any site can be involved.

Other varietes
(1) *Guttate form* consisting of very white round drop-like atrophic macules. The lesions may become larger by coalescence. (2) *Coup de sabre*, which presents itself as a wide sabre-shaped band extending from the forehead towards the vertex, lying close to the median line.

It may be associated with epilepsy and atrophy of one side of the face.

COURSE

The lesions usually slowly resolve.

TREATMENT

Intralesional steroids are worth using in these cases.

Systemic or Progressive Scleroderma

This is a rare, very serious, chronic condition, characterized by the progressive induration and atrophy of connective tissue all over the body. It commonly affects women between 30 and 50, although no age or sex is exempt. The most favoured cause is a disturbance of immunological mechanisms.

CLINICAL FEATURES

The onset is insidious. The skin changes are usually preceded by signs of Raynaud's phenomenon. The skin becomes hard and stiff and movements become severely restricted. The face, hands, and forearms are first attacked, and soon the face is contracted and immobile, the lips thin and pinched and the chin puckered. Mastication becomes very difficult, and the hands cannot be closed into a fist, and later they are useless. Trophic ulcerations and gangrene are common terminal sequelae. Systemic changes follow, such as severe dysphagia, dyspnoea, and cardiac insufficiency. Hypergammaglobulinaemia is present.

COURSE

The spread varies in rate, but is relentless. The survival rate is 20 years or more. Remission is rare. Death is commonly due to renal or heart failure.

DIAGNOSIS

This is made by the characteristic contracted facies, and the restricted movements.

Raynaud's disease is characterized by paroxysmal attacks of ischaemia, with numbness and paleness. *Syringomyelia* presents dissociated areas of anaesthesia.

TREATMENT

Steroids often are beneficial in the early stages of the disease.

Physiotherapy and exercises are essential in an effort to postpone contractions. Cold is to be avoided, and patients should, if possible, live in a warm climate, but there is no treatment which can guarantee permanent relief.

Dermatomyositis

This is an acute, subacute, or chronic disorder characterized by dermatitis of various types, oedema, muscular pains, non-suppurative inflammation, and degeneration of the muscles.

The cause is unknown, but its occasional association with S.L.E., rheumatoid arthritis and systemic sclerosis suggests a common aetiology. Both sexes are equally affected and no age is exempt but it is commonest in the fifth decade. It is an uncommon condition.

CLINICAL FEATURES

The onset is insidious or sudden, and may follow an infection. Puffiness of the face develops and, notably, of the eyelids and malar area. The puffiness recedes leaving a reticulated telangiectatic erythema, and an appearance of atrophy. Muscular pain and tenderness vary, and any muscle may be affected. The ESR is high.

Association with carcinoma of various organs is not uncommon, and is the usual cause of death.

DIAGNOSIS

This is confirmed by the finding of a raised serum creatine kinase, by abnormal potentials on electromyography or by muscle biopsy. vary, and any muscle may be affected.

Carcinoma of various organs is not uncommon, and is the usual cause of death.

TREATMENT

Rest, but not absolute bed-rest except in the acute phase, and high calorie diets. Steroids may suppress the disease. Physiotherapy may help prevent contractures.

PROGNOSIS

The course is unpredictable. Some patients die within a few weeks to a few years of onset. Others recover, or become chronic cases indefinitely.

Reiter's Disease

The cause of this condition is unknown. The most constant features are polyarthritis and non-gonococcal urethritis with conjunctivitis or iritis in about a half of all patients. It may be seen in association with venereally acquired urethritis or as a complication of dysentery or non-specific diarrhoea.

CLINICAL FEATURES

Lesions of the skin and mucous membranes are found in some patients and the commonest site to be affected is the penis (about 25 per cent of all cases). Shallow, circular, red erosions appear on the mucous membrane of the glans and prepuce ('circinate balanitis'). If the patient is circumcised the lesions tend to coalesce and brownish 'keratodermic' crusts may develop.

Similar erosive lesions are found on the mucous membrane of the mouth, tongue and oropharynx in about 15 per cent of patients. On occasion a severe stomatitis may develop though in general it is most unusual for mucous membrane lesions to cause symptoms. Their presence should always be sought therefore in any case of arthritis where the aetiology is not clear.

The characteristic lesions of the skin, 'keratoderma blenorrhagica' are seen in about 10 per cent of patients and usually in those most severely affected. The commonest site where the first lesions appear is the soles of the feet (Plate 32). They appear as dull brownish red macules which rapidly progress through vesiculation to apparent pustulation. These 'pustules' may run together to form large lesions 3 to 5 cm in diameter. Eventually keratinization begins and layers of yellowish brown scale accumulate often producing crusted limpet-like masses. In severely affected patients lesions may be found anywhere on the body. Toe and fingernails may be affected with thickening, ridging and opacity of the nails. In such severe cases the eruption may persist for many months. In the type of case most commonly seen the lesions are restricted to the feet and clear in a few weeks or months.

TREATMENT

Circinate balanitis rarely requires treatment though severe cases are helped by local application of ½ per cent steroid creams. Extensive keratoderma will often respond to oral steroids though the response of the inflamed joints is frequently disappointing.

Skin conditions related to systemic diseases of known aetiology

Many skin diseases are associated with, or provoked by conditions in other organs, and those predominantly concerned are the endocrine glands.

The skin changes associated with hyper- and hypo-pigmentation are well documented in text-books on general medicine, as well as acromegaly and Cushing's syndrome in the case of pituitary disorders. In disorders associated with the pancreas, apart from jaundice, the skin produces remarkably few changes.

Intestinal diseases, such as ulcerative colitis, may cause urticaria, leg ulcers, and erythema nodosum.

Renal disorders may be associated with neurofibromatosis, systemic lupus erythematosus, scleroderma, anaphylactoid purpura and erythema multiforme, as well as pruritus, which is a classical symptom of uraemia.

Conditions complicating malignancy in other organs are dealt with on page 252.

CHAPTER 18

Diseases of the Appendages

Acne: Seborrhoea: Sebaceous Cysts: Hyperidrosis:
Cheilitis: Perlèche: Stomatitis: Peri-Oral Dermatitis:
Leucoplakia: Ringworm of Nails: Paronychia: Ingrowing Nail:
Hypertrophy of Nail: Secondary Nail Conditions: Alopecia:
Hirsuties: Greying of Hair: Ingrowing Hairs: Monilethrix

SEBACEOUS GLANDS

Acne Vulgaris

This is a chronic inflammatory disease, characterized by comedones (blackheads), papules, pustules, and sometimes cysts, involving the sebaceous follicles and glands. Obstruction of the pilo-sebaceous canal, increased sebum production, skin surface lipid changes, and bacterial involvement of the follicles, appear to be important factors, and related to each other.

CAUSE
The exact cause is unknown.

Age
Any time after puberty until the age of 30.

Heredity
There appears to be greater tendency for acne to develop when there is a familial history of the disease.

Season and Climate
Acne is more common in winter, and in temperate zones.

Hormones
The age of onset of acne coincides with a momentous hormonal revolution and sebaceous gland activity is mediated by androgens.

PATHOLOGY

Examination of a comedo shows that it is composed of sebum, and horny and uncornified cells, lying in a pilo-sebaceous follicle. The black tip of the comedo is due to melanin. The comedo is surrounded by an inflammatory infiltrate of varying intensity which accounts for the redness around the lesion. When pustular lesions are present, pus cells are found, sometimes with the formation of small abscesses, and disintegration of the follicle.

CLINICAL FEATURES

There are no symptoms: only those of embarrassment which may be latent unless the patient is questioned on the point. This is the result of bad medical or parental advice, which consists mainly of stating that acne is a normal event in the process of growing up, and that the spots will disappear with time. Both statements are to a certain extent true, but they do not invalidate the necessity for energetic treatment which will hasten recovery.

The onset is gradual. The lesions consist of comedones, papules, and pustules, and occasionally cysts. They are found on the face (Fig. 53), chest and back, and back of the neck. In number they vary from a few to hundreds; the skin of the acne patient is often greasy, and the complexion, brunette. Dandruff is commonly present in varying degrees.

Other varieties

Excoriated acne occurs as a result of neurotic and intensive picking of lesions, and is usually seen in females. It is best treated by reassurance, and recommending a masking cream such as Covermark or Erase. This reduces the tendency to pick the lesions.

Infantile acne occurs in babies during the first year, and 80 per cent are males. Erythromycin 250 mg b.d. for 2–3 months may be given in some cases.

Acne keloid is a chronic staphylococcal infection of the hair follicles of the back of the neck of men, which result in the formation of unsightly hypertrophic scars. It is best treated by intralesional hydrocortisone.

Acne conglobata is a rare variant of acne, characterized by the formation of abscesses, sinuses, and scars.

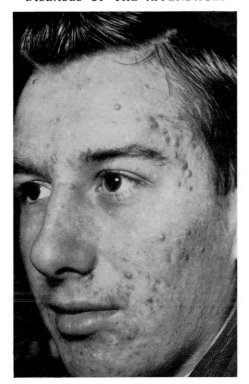

FIG. 53. Acne vulgaris.

Iatrogenic acne. Acne can be provoked or initiated by such drugs as oral steroids, ACTH, iodides, or bromides.

Occupational acne is not a variety of acne vulgaris, but produces similar lesions, as a result of the person working in contact with oils, waxes, tars, chlornaphthalenes, or asbestos.

DIAGNOSIS

This is usually quite simple. *Rosacea* may imitate acne vulgaris to a certain extent, but there are no comedones, the condition is usually symmetrical, involving the face; the chest and back are rarely involved, and it occurs after the age of 30. *Peri-oral dermatitis* is seen mostly in females, characterized by small, itchy papules and pustules round the mouth. It responds to oxytetracycline 250 mg tablets b.d. for 2–3 months, and hydrocortisone cream b.d.

TREATMENT

An optimistic approach must be made with whatever form of treatment is employed. Plenty of rest, exercise and sleep should be emphasized, advice which young people often find difficult to follow. Frequent washing of the face, i.e. at least four times a day, should be encouraged with soap and warm water. When the eating of chocolates and fatty foods appears to produce more lesions, these foods must be avoided. Squeezing and picking of the lesions are not helpful. Contrary to the belief of some, marriage does not cure acne.

External
Sulphur causes mild peeling of the skin, and is best used in a lotion, as a cream is redundant to any already greasy skin. Sulphurated potash and zinc lotion B.N.F. is the most favoured of sulphur-containing lotions. The peeling encourages removal of the superficial part of the comedo. Benzoyl peroxide lotion, and topical vitamin A (retinoic acid) may be tried, but may irritate the skin.

There is little place for the use of topical corticosteroids in acne, and it may be exacerbated by the use of fluorinated steroids.

Brasivol ointment, which consists of finely-ground aluminium oxide in an emulsifying base, is useful in some cases as a mild abrasive. A more satisfactory method of gently and temporarily exfoliating the skin is by ultra-violet radiation (u.v.r.). Exposures producing a 2nd degree erythema may be given twice a week. U.V.R. is particularly helpful in brunettes, but on blonde skins may produce ill-timed discomfort and therefore should be used with caution.

CO_2 slush, which consists of ground CO_2 snow mixed with acetone, can be swabbed over the affected areas, and this also produces a peeling effect.

X-rays in appropriate doses cause reduction in the size and activity of the sebaceous gland, and therefore may be employed in carefully selected cases of those over the age of 17. Many dermatologists are opposed to this form of therapy.

X-rays do not remove blackheads. This is best done by means of a comedo expressor. This is a spoon-handled object, with a hole in it. When pressed on the spot, the comedo exudes through the orifice. Dermabrasion is a little-used method of planing skin which is scarred; it is performed with a revolving burr, resembling a dentist's drill. The cosmetic results do not justify its use.

Internal

The oxytetracycline group of drugs are the most useful form of internal treatment. It leads to a decrease in the number of Coryne-bacteria acnes, and surface lipid free fatty acids. In most cases oxytetracyclines such as Imperacin, or Clinimycin in a dosage of 250 mg three times daily for a week, an hour before meals, and subsequently twice daily, for many weeks or months, is the only form of treatment which maintains a reasonable and presentable appearance. Erythromycin may be used as an alternative.

Hormones can be used in cases where there seems to be a particular relationship of the appearance of lesions to the menstrual cycle. The contraceptive pill often produces good results, and where parents are opposed to its use, they may accept it when it is explained that only a short course of 3–4 months will be required. A double daily dose may have to be given, and a product containing a non-androgenic progestin should be prescribed.

There is evidence that prednisone may help in selected cases of severe acne, when other measures fail. There is no doubt that intra-lesional hydrocortisone is often beneficial for large cystic lesions.

PROGNOSIS

All patients can be improved. 90 per cent should be cured except for the appearance of an occasional lesion, but this depends on the confidence of the patient in the treatment, and the doctor's ability to inspire it. Furthermore, the patient should accept the fact that a cure will take several months.

Seborrhoea

This term implies that there is an increased flow of sebum.

It is an inborn and common characteristic of many people, and produces excessive oiliness of the skin, particularly of the nose and central areas of the face, whose follicles tend to gape.

The hair becomes greasy, and frequent shampooing allays symptoms for only a day or two. The condition usually occurs at puberty at lasts as a post-pubertal state for a few years; it occasionally persists indefinitely.

Treatment consists of shampoos used two or three times a week, such as Genisol or Polytar, followed by the application of salicylic acid lotion B.P.C., or Dermovate scalp lotion.

Sebaceous Cysts

These are smooth, round, globular, cutaneous or subcutaneous tumours which arise from the sebaceous glands, and are found on the face, neck, scalp, back and genitalia. They may be single, or multiple (pilar cysts).

CAUSE
Unknown. Pilar cysts are often hereditary.

PATHOLOGY
The cyst contains cheesy, smelly material, consisting of masses of degenerating and disintegrating epithelial cells. It is encapsulated by fibrous connective tissue. The pathology of the pilar cysts differs.

CLINICAL FEATURES
The size of the tumour varies from a pea to an orange or larger. The surface is smooth and shiny. On palpation they feel soft and doughy, or firm. Number: one or several.

Malignant change is very rare.

TREATMENT
Excision, to include the epithelial wall, otherwise the cyst will probably reform.

SWEAT GLANDS

Sweat glands occur all over the body, except on the margins of the lips, the glans penis, and the inner surface of the prepuce. They are most numerous on the palms and soles. For fuller details, see Chapter 1, p. 3.

Hyperidrosis

This means an excessive production of sweat. It may be idiopathic, or symptomatic of other conditions, generalized or localized, and bilaterally or unilaterally distributed.

CAUSE

When symptomatic it may be due to hyperthyroidism, diabetes mellitus, tuberculosis, malaria, or organic disease of the central nervous system. Anxiety states and neuroses cause hyperidrosis, and many patients suffer from it in the presence of a doctor. It is also provoked by warmth, alcohol, and aspirin. In some cases, it is a familial disorder.

CLINICAL FEATURES

The patient may complain of intense discomfort from excessive sweating of the hands, feet or axillae, so much so in some cases that ability to work is impaired.

The skin of the palms and soles becomes thickened and develops a bluish-grey colour. Nail deformities may occur.

TREATMENT

Any underlying cause must be treated. When functional, the following therapies may be tried:

1. Wear only cotton socks and change daily. The same applies to underwear, when necessary. Hair should be cut short in the axillae when they are affected.

2. Formaldehyde 2 per cent in water, dabbed on 2 or 3 times a week, not forgetting that formaldehyde is capable on occasion of causing dermatitis.

3. Hexametaphosphate 5 per cent in water, applied daily.

4. Sympathectomy is sometimes effective for severe hyperidrosis of the palms, but not for the soles. Some degree of Horner's syndrome occurs as a side effect of the operation in a considerable proportion of cases.

Local resection of the sweat glands for axillary hyperidrosis is carried out by a plastic surgeon; sweating is reduced by 70 per cent.

5. For axillary hyperidrosis, the hair should be kept shaven, and anti-perspirant lotions used. They usually contain aluminium salts, and should only be applied when the axillae are dry.

6. X-rays should not be used.

MUCOUS MEMBRANES

Introduction

This section deals only with those mucous membranes which are adjacent to the skin, namely, the oral, nasal and conjunctival, the penile, vulvar, vaginal and anal.

Although they have neither a horny layer, hairs, nor sweat glands (in the mouth especially, however, there are mucous glands), the mucous membranes are subject to a great many disorders to which the skin is also liable and in the same way; they are, for example, prone to allergic, infective and malignant processes.

In quite a number of skin conditions, mucous membrane lesions co-exist, and therefore examination of these surfaces must not be omitted. Sometimes they will enable one to confirm an otherwise difficult differential diagnosis.

It is profitable to acquire the habit of examining the mouth, in the general examination of a case, so that one does not omit the examination when a disease with which oral lesions are associated presents itself. Even when oral lesions exist, recognition is not always straightforward, for the uncornified fragile mucous membrane is soon broken and macerated by the evolution of the lesion. It is important, therefore, to look for the early unaltered lesion.

Oral examination refers to the lips, tongue, palate and gums. Lesions on these areas may be part of a disease localized to the mucous membranes; they may also exist in the presence of skin lesions; and they may be the forerunners of a skin eruption. This precept also applies to mucous membrane lesions in other sites, although in other sites lesions are, as a rule, more likely to exist without skin lesions.

The lesions associated with skin diseases are described under the named disease. They are lichen planus, syphilis, erythema multiforme and pemphigus. Other less common diseases are also associated with oral lesions.

ORAL LESIONS

The Lips

Cheilitis

This means inflammation of the lips, and is characterized by scaling, crusting, and fissuring.

CAUSE

Chemical agents. Lipsticks, toothpastes and mouthwashes.
Physical agents. Sunlight sensitivity.
Trauma. Habitual licking of the lips.
Infections. Candidiasis is the usual cause.
Secondary to skin conditions, such as seborrhoeic dermatitis, or atopic dermatitis.

TREATMENT

Removal and/or treatment of the cause. Local steroids always help except in the case of candidiasis, when nystatin cream should be applied.

Perlèche

This is an inflammatory condition at the junctures where the lips meet, and is characterized by fissuring, maceration and crusting of the area.

CAUSE

Candida albicans, streptococcal or staphylococcal infection. These may be transmitted directly, or by the communal use of cups and towels, in closed communities such as schools. Infection may also develop in people with badly fitting dentures, which may alter the angle where the lips meet, thus creating a warm moist folded area of skin suitable for the growth of organisms.

TREATMENT

Avoid communal use of cups and towels. Faulty dentures should be corrected. Apply a steroid ointment combined with an antibiotic, or nystatin ointment when *Candida albicans* is present.

Peri-oral dermatitis is a condition in which small red macules, papules or pustules surround the mouth. It may extend to involve the cheeks, chin and forehead. It may be idiopathic or due to prolonged application of a steroid preparation. Oxytetracycline 250 mg b.d. for 2 months is usually effective.

Herpes simplex (see p. 154).

Chronic infections: (1) extragenital chancre; (2) lepromatous leprosy; (3) sarcoidosis.

The Mouth

Aphthous Stomatitis

This is a recurrent vesicular condition of the mouth.

CAUSE

This is unknown. Some cases are associated with emotional stress, others with gastrointestinal disturbances.

CLINICAL FEATURES

An extremely sore mouth, which induces apprehension regarding eating and drinking, because this accentuates the soreness.

The onset is sudden. Lesions are vesicular. They are very small, yellowish, and soon ulcerate. They are found on the side of the tongue, or its under-surface, on the inner surface of the lips and the gums. Occasionally the genitalia are affected.

COURSE

Lesions are recurrent, taking about 2 weeks to heal. The intervals between attacks vary from years to weeks.

DIAGNOSIS

Candidiasis is excluded by the absence of organisms, and the absence of foetor, fever and lymphadenopathy precludes Vincent's angina.

TREATMENT

There is nothing specific. Hot food and drink, which worsens the condition, must be avoided. Mouth-washes and the application of 1 per cent silver nitrate may help. Corlan pellets dissolved in the mouth may be soothing. Oxytetracycline oral suspension (Terramycin) 250 mg (5 ml) given 4 times daily for 5–7 days is often beneficial. It is held in the mouth for 2 minutes, then swallowed. Nothing should be eaten for 1 hour after each dose.

Leucoplakia

This condition is characterized by white patches on the lips and on any of the mucous membranes of the body. It is a potentially malignant disease.

CAUSE

This is unknown, except when syphilis is present.

Predisposing factors

Any form of chronic irritation such as smoking or jagged teeth may produce oral lesions. Blond-skinned people are more liable to suffer, whilst males far outnumber females. The commonest age is between 40 and 70.

CLINICAL FEATURES

At the onset there is slight irritation of the area, associated with marked sensitivity to hot and spicy foods and drinks. The lesions are flat at the onset, later becoming slightly raised. They may be very small, or the size of a sixpence, or larger. They vary in shape, being usually roughly round, but may appear as streaks, bands or nodules. They are always well defined, although the edge is irregular. The surface is flat and smooth and, as the name implies, the lesions are white. To the touch, they are somewhat rough, and may feel thickened. They are most commonly found on the dorsum and lateral sulci of the tongue, the inner surfaces of the cheeks along the interdental line, and the gums, especially at the angle of the jaw.

On the female genitalia, the clitoris, the inner surfaces of the labia and the perineum are most commonly affected; in the male, the glans penis occasionally. When lesions are present on the genitalia, itching may be very severe, although intermittent.

COURSE

When the condition affects the mouth, cessation of smoking, attention to teeth or dentures, and the avoidance of stimulating food and drink, usually result in the disappearance of the lesions. Should no improvement occur within two months, surgical treatment must be given.

Vulval lesions become malignant in 5 per cent of cases, and should therefore always be biopsied.

DIAGNOSIS

This is made by the characteristic whiteness, and the irregular and well-defined lesions. *Syphilis* can be excluded by other signs of the disease, and *lichen planus* by lesions characteristic of that disease found elsewhere in the body.

TREATMENT

Cauterization or excision of oral lesions is best, whilst vulvectomy may be necessary for vulval lesions.

NAILS

The anatomy and pathology of the nails, and other aspects, are considered in Chapter 1.

Nail affections may be primary, or secondary to other conditions, both dermatological and non-dermatological.

PRIMARY CONDITIONS

1. Ringworm

This and other fungal infections of the nails are dealt with in Chapter 10.

2. Paronychia

This is an acute or subacute inflammation of the peri-ungual tissues of one or more nails (Fig. 54).

CAUSE

Usually *Candida albicans*, occasionally streptococci or staphylococci.

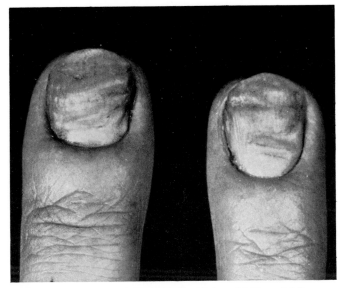

Fig. 54. Paronychia showing bolstering of the nail-folds, and deformity of the nails (Institute of Dermatology, University of London).

Sex
Women more often affected than men.

Occupation
Bar-work, laundry-work, kitchen-work, manicuring; for maceration of the skin due to excessive immersion in liquids facilitates the entry of organisms under the nail-fold.

CLINICAL FEATURES
Pain localized to the peri-ungual tissues. The peri-ungual tissues of one or more digits is swollen, red, macerated, and painful to the touch. The middle finger is most commonly affected first. Gentle pressure on the bolstered nail-fold may result in the expression of a bead of pus.

TREATMENT

The most important factor is to keep the finger dry. If no organisms can be cultured, Nystan ointment or Fungilin lotion should first be used. It is gently inserted on a finely pared, square-ended orange stick, under the nailfold, three times daily. Should no improvement occur after 2 to 3 weeks, eusol lotion, or Penotrane jelly, may be applied in the same way. Avulsion of the nail is not recommended.

PROGNOSIS

Most cases clear up in 6–10 weeks, but recurrences are not un-common. These can be minimized by the avoidance of excessive washing, and protecting the finger with a rubber stall whilst following an occupation demanding immersion in liquids.

3. Ingrowing Nail

In this condition the lateral border of the toenail grows into the surrounding soft tissues.

CAUSE

Tight shoes, usually.

TREATMENT

Spacious shoes. Also cut a V into the middle of the free edge of the nail. Relief of pain may be obtained by the daily application of cold Kaolin ointment on lint.

4. Hypertrophy of the Nail (Onychogryphosis)

The toe-nails become enormous, deformed and filthy, the condition is frequently due to neglect and badly fitting shoes. It is common in vagrants.

SECONDARY CONDITIONS

1. Clubbing of the Fingers

Known also as Hippocratic fingers, hypertrophy of the nail bed results in enlargement and curving in both directions of the finger and/or toe nails, with loss of the angle at the base of the nail.

They are due, among other causes, to chronic lung diseases, such as bronchiectasis and carcinoma of the lung, chronic heart disease, such as cyanotic congenital heart disease, or sub-acute bacterial endocarditis, and occasionally chronic gastro-intestinal disease, for example Crohn's. In about 10 per cent of cases the cause is familial.

2. Spoon-shaped Nails, or Koilonychia

May be congenital in origin, or due to the Plummer-Vinson syndrome. Occasionally they have been noted in coronary artery disease, syphilis, and in users of strong alkalis. The nails are so shaped that if a drop of water is placed on them it will not roll off.

3. Leuconychia

These are white spots or streaks on the nails, and are usually congenital or due to trauma. They may also appear spontaneously, as a result of air in the nail.

4. Brittleness of the Nails

May be congenital or acquired. When acquired, it is due to detergents, nail polish or polish removers, myxoedema, or old age.

5. Shedding of Nails

This sometimes accompanies alopecia areata, and is a minor complication of infectious fevers, such as typhoid and meningitis. The nails ultimately grow again, except in severe peripheral vascular disease.

6. Pigmentation of the Nails

May be due to the use of potassium permanganate as an antiseptic finger bath, or the taking of phenolphthalein, a constituent of some laxatives, or mepacrine which is used in cases of chronic lupus erythematosus and malaria.

7. Nail Changes in Skin Diseases

These are dealt with elsewhere in the description of the disease but a summary is given in Table 4.

TABLE 4

Nail changes which may occur, singly or severally in some skin diseases

PSORIASIS	'Thimble pitting', yellowish discoloration, subungual accumulation of horny material
ECZEMA	Irregularity, ridging
CHRONIC PARONYCHIA	Distortion and ridging
ALOPECIA AREATA	Temporary arrest of growth, or fall
ICHTHYOSIS	Discoloration, subungual thickening
LICHEN PLANUS	Discoloration, ridging, and shedding

HAIR

The anatomy, function and other aspects of the hair, are dealt with in Chapter 1.

ALOPECIA

Alopecia, or baldness, may be congenital or acquired, congenital baldness being very uncommon. Consideration of any form of alopecia must embrace all the hairy areas of the body. The scalp is most commonly affected, but involvement of the groins, beard, axillae, and pubes must be borne in mind.

Congenital Alopecia

This may be complete, permanent, and generalized, or variations of these states may occur. For example, there may be complete or partial alopecia followed later by the development of normal growth.

Congenital alopecia is frequently associated with abnormal growth, or absence of teeth or nails, and skin irregularities. It is worth remembering that where one congenital anomaly occurs, others frequently exist in other organs and tissues.

CAUSE
Unknown.

Sex
The condition is more common in men.

Heredity
More often than not, no relevant history can be elicited.

Treatment
None effective.

Prognosis
This is impossible to forecast, and as a rule no growth should be expected.

Acquired Alopecia

Common Baldness
This is the commonest form of baldness, and accounts for at least 95 per cent of all cases.

CAUSE
Unknown.

Theories
The most popular current theories vacillate between genetic, hormonal, or ageing factors as being responsible, severally or singly.

Sex
Men far outnumber women, as is obvious from daily observation.

CLINICAL FEATURES
The onset is gradual. The baldness is never scattered, and pursues a well-recognized course, producing one of the common types of male

baldness. Recession may occur in the fronto-parietal areas, or on the crown of the head, or on both regions simultaneously. The rate of hair-fall varies in each person, and cannot be anticipated.

DIAGNOSIS

This is made by the pattern of recession, and the absence of broken hairs (see alopecia areata).

TREATMENT

There is no effective prophylactic or curative treatment known. Promises made by quack hair-restorers are baseless.

Alopecia Areata

This form of alopecia is characterized by a loss of hair in round or oval, well-defined patches, without inflammation.

CAUSE
Unknown.

Sex
Both sexes are equally affected.

Age
Any age may be affected, but the commonest is childhood. At least 20 per cent occur before the age of ten.

Heredity
It has often occurred in several members of a family. There are also reports of identical cases in twins. An hereditary history in at least 20 per cent of a series of cases is not unusual.

Psychological Factors
Much has been written in favour of and against the involvement of such factors in alopecia areata. There are many cases of the condition being coincidental, for example, with bereavements of a close relation, the ordeals of domestic strife, or the unfulfilment of ambition; there are also many cases with no apparent emotional disturbance whatsoever, so that it is difficult to be dogmatic. Each case must be judged on its merits.

Other theories
Virus infections and hormonal disturbances have been blamed, but such assumptions have yet to be proven.

CLINICAL FEATURES

There are no symptoms.

The onset is nearly always sudden. In some cases, an area may become completely bald overnight, the patient finding a cluster of hairs on the pillow. In other cases, baldness develops over the course of a few days. The size of the area varies from that of a sixpence to the palm of the hand, or larger (Fig. 55). Their shape is generally

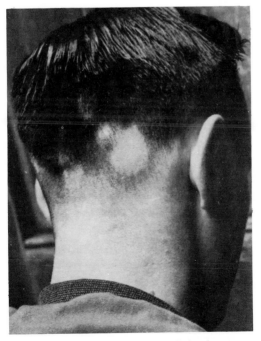

FIG. 55. Alopecia areata. Partial scalp involvement.

round, but may be oval, or very irregular due to coalescence of patches. The surface of the scalp is white, soft, and smooth; and close examination will reveal very short broken stumps of hair, which are clearly thicker at the top than at the skin surface, illustrating a characteristic feature of the disease, namely exclamation-mark hair, thus, !. When they disappear, arrest of the balding process has begun. Any site on the scalp may be involved. Any hairs remaining may be easily removed, and whilst the patch is active, long hairs at the edge are easily pulled out with their shiny root-sheaths. Once activity ceases, the hairs are firm. The eyebrows, beard, moustache and eyelashes are other areas which may be involved. The number of patches ranges from one to many.

COURSE

Regrowth is not a certainty, but usual. As regrowth occurs, the hairs appear as soft down, and are soon replaced by thicker white hairs, which are later replaced again by pigmented normal hairs. During these phases, a piebald appearance may be expected.

Variations of Alopecia

(i) *Alopecia totalis:* signifies loss of hair over the entire scalp (Fig. 56).
(ii) *Alopecia universalis:* loss of hair over the entire body.
(iii) *Diffuse alopecia:* this occurs on the scalp. It may occur in young women, and last for several months to 2 years: it may be caused by oral contraceptives: it may follow a severe illness, e.g. meningitis, typhoid fever.
(iv) *Traction alopecia:* is found on the frontal and occipital areas, as a result of the hair being pulled when the 'pony tail' style is worn, or when pulled by the use of tight curlers.

TREATMENT

Although there is nothing specific some mild counter-irritant should be given, and attention paid to the general health of the patient.

External

Painting the area with 1 or 2 per cent phenol by means of a worn toothbrush, every 2 days, is sometimes useful, as the patient is usually anxious to have something to apply. One injection of a steroid preparation into small patches is often enough to initiate

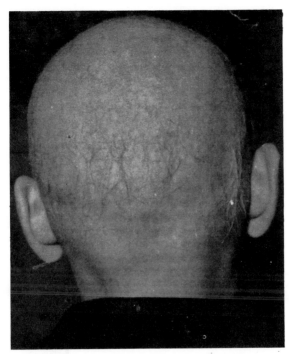

FIG. 56. Alopecia areata. Total scalp involvement.

regrowth, at times more than one injection may be necessary. (Steroids are useless for male pattern baldness.)

Internal
Tonics and iron when indicated may be helpful.

DIAGNOSIS
This is made by the history of sudden hair fall in patches, the scalp being normal except for exclamation-mark and loose hairs.

PROGNOSIS

The younger the patient the better the outlook. The older patient is always very anxious concerning regrowth and the possibility of complete baldness, and therefore the prognosis often depends to a large extent on the enthusiasm and confidence of the doctor. Intralesional steroids have greatly improved the prognosis, although they are hardly justified in children.

Hirsuties

Hirsuties is also known by the term hypertrichosis, both words signifying superfluous hair. This is found on areas which naturally have downy hair. It may be congenital or acquired.

Sex

It is found equally in both sexes, but it is women who seek medical advice because of its embarrassment to them.

Race

There is a tendency for the condition to be more common amongst Jews, Negroes and Spaniards.

Hormonal disturbances

Pregnancy is sometimes accompanied by sudden hirsuties, which is usually transitory. The menopause is also sometimes associated with the gradual appearance of superfluous hair, which is, however, permanent.

Other conditions, such as Cushing's syndrome, the adreno-genital syndrome, acromegaly, tumours of the pineal gland, and hyperthyroidism must also be considered as causes of hirsuties.

Psychological factors

Anorexia nervosa is always accompanied by hirsuties of the downy type, although some coarse hairs may be seen.

Drugs

Steroids may produce hirsuties.

CLINICAL FEATURES

In women, mental distress is the predominant feature.

(a) *Congenital type.* In severe cases, the entire body and face may be covered with hair. Persons so afflicted may earn a living working in travelling circuses. A lock of hair confined to the lumbo-sacral area may be associated with spina bifida. Other anomalies distributed on small areas of the body may be found. Dental defects may be found with the localized variety of hirsuties.

(b) *Acquired type.* Where there is no obvious cause, in the case of a healthy woman, the superfluous hair is always localized, and found on the beard area. Psychoses may develop.

When hirsuties is due to a primary condition, for example, Cushing's syndrome, that condition will clearly declare itself as the cause.

In children, transient hirsuties may be seen, varying in magnitude and distribution, in such conditions as tuberculosis, coeliac disease, malnutrition or pink disease.

TREATMENT

Temporary removal can be obtained by the judicious use of a pumice stone, by shaving, or better still, by waxes. The wax is applied soft and warm, and when cool is rapidly removed pulling with it attached hairs. This operation is repeated every 3 or 4 weeks. None of these methods increases hair growth. For less exuberant hirsuties, bleaching by means of hydrogen peroxide with cotton wool once or twice a week disguises the condition.

Permanent removal is obtained by using a diathermy needle, which is inserted into the hair follicle.

ANOMALIES OF HAIR-GROWTH

Some of the many anomalies are worth mentioning.

1. Greying of the hair

This is very common, and the cause is unknown. A familial tendency is probably the commonest factor.

2. Ingrowing hairs, or pili incarnati

These hairs turn round and re-enter the skin, after surfacing. The beard area is commonly affected; when the eyelashes are concerned, conjunctivitis may occur as the hair is in the process of turning on itself. Growing a beard is sometimes effective in training the hair to grow outwards. For eyelashes, epilation should be used.

3. Monilethrix

A congenital and hereditary condition, characterized by dull, thin brittle hair on the scalp, with beaded swellings of the hair shaft. Both sexes are affected. Normal growth sometimes occurs spontaneously at puberty.

CHAPTER 19

Tumours

Seborrhoeic Warts: Keloid: Fibroma: Neurofibroma:
Solar Keratosis: Granuloma Pyogenicum: Kerato-Acanthoma:
Basal Cell Carcinoma: Squamous Cell Carcinoma: Paget's
Disease of Nipple: Malignant Melanoma: Hodgkin's Disease:
Leukaemia: Metastatic Carcinoma: Skin Changes related to
Internal Cancer

Introduction

A tumour is a mass, and in the lay mind is *ipso facto* considered to be malignant.

Tumours of the skin, like tumours of any other tissue, can, of course, be benign or malignant.

By definition, their characteristics in the skin vary enormously, being soft or hard, freely mobile or fixed to the surrounding tissue, being raised above the skin surface or situated deep in it, whilst their shape and size know no uniformity.

The commonest malignant conditions of the skin are the basal cell and the squamous cell carcinoma, and the former is more prevalent than the latter. But by and large, masses in or on the skin, in this country, are more often benign than malignant.

The most heartening feature of the basal cell carcinoma is that it very, very rarely spreads systematically through the body, although the squamous cell carcinoma will do so if not dealt with early enough.

Some benign tumours, such as haemangiomata or birthmarks, and cellular naevi or moles, are dealt with in Chapter 20.

BENIGN TUMOURS

Seborrhoeic Warts (Senile Warts)

The title is misleading, for these lesions are not warts in the sense that they are caused by a virus, nor are they, therefore, infectious (the cause is unknown), but in appearance they are what one recognizes as warty. Nor are they associated with seborrhoea. And again, senility is not an essential condition for their existence. Such is the confusion of nomenclature. Although they are commonly found in old people, they may develop at the age of forty. Nevertheless, seborrhoeic is a better word to use than senile in the patient's hearing.

PATHOLOGY

Hyperkeratosis, acanthosis and papillomatosis are apparent, and the basal layer is notably hyperpigmented. The pigmentation varies in density, which accounts for the different shades of brown of the clinical lesion.

CLINICAL FEATURES

The lesions are papular, the size varying from 1–2 cm. in diameter. They are round or oval, the surface is rough and flat, and their colour varies from light to dark brown (Plate 33). The commonest site is the trunk, and they also occur on the temples and elsewhere. Sometimes a few exist, at other times they are scattered haphazardly over the trunk.

DIAGNOSIS

They must be distinguished from pigmented moles which are very smooth, well defined, and appear earlier in life.

TREATMENT

Curetting followed by cauterization, or cauterization alone.

Keloid

This is a firm, irregularly-shaped tumour, which may be smooth or ridged, occurring generally on the area of a scar or a previous injury.

CAUSE

(a) An individual predisposition.
(b) A racial predisposition, especially in Negroes.
(c) A regional susceptibility, in that keloids commonly occur in areas where an injury crosses normal flexion creases.

(d) Trauma, which, however slight, may initiate the formation of a keloid in susceptible people.

PATHOLOGY

The collagenous tissue of the dermis is enormously increased and obliterates the elastic tissue and, partially, the blood vessels in the area. This increase of collagen accounts for the tumour formation.

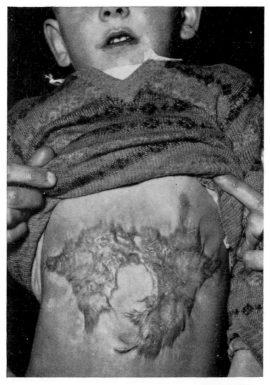

FIG. 57. Keloid, which followed a burn from boiling water.

CLINICAL FEATURES

The onset is gradual. The lesions are smooth or ridged swellings.
Their size varies from a pip to a plate (Fig. 57), and any kind of
shape may develop, such as a cord, lozenge or spider. The surface
is glossy and smooth, and the colour which is at first red, becomes
pink, and finally white with age. Any site may be affected.

TREATMENT

Intralesional hydrocortisone in young lesions is often most effective.
About two to six injections at weekly intervals usually suffice.

X-ray therapy followed by excision, in some hands, has also proved
to be curative.

Old lesions usually resist all forms of treatment.

Fibroma

This is a hard, painless, well-defined nodule, usually found on the
extremities, in adults. In some cases, multiple lesions exist. Pedunculated lesions may be seen on the genitalia.

PATHOLOGY

Two types exist; in one, the chief cells are histiocytes, in the other
fibroblasts. The lesion is well defined but does not have a capsule.
The clear definition is due to a band of normal collagen. The lesion
contains innumerable histiocytes, which contain lipoids, and giant
cells are also present.

CLINICAL FEATURES

The onset is quite rapid. The lesion becomes akin to an acorn's nut,
shiny and firm, with epidermis very adherent to it.

TREATMENT

Excision, if required.

Neurofibroma

This condition is characterized by numerous, flabby, flesh-coloured
or brownish pedunculated tumours, and brown macules (Fig. 58).

There are 3 types:

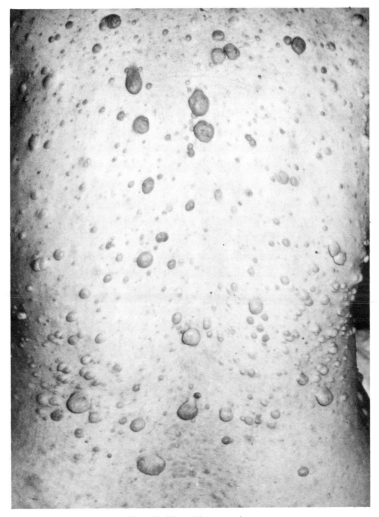

FIG. 58. Neurofibromatosis.

(i) Superficial, which is the type most commonly seen in skin clinics.

(ii) Deep, where the lesions are attached to the peripheral parts of nerve trunks.

(iii) Multiple neurofibromatosis, or von Recklinghausen's disease.

PATHOLOGY

The tumour is comparatively acellular, and is composed of wavy bundles of fibroblastic cells, with long thin nuclei separated by loose connective tissue, in which groups of nerve fibres are easily visible.

CLINICAL FEATURES

(1) Superficial type: these are pin-head in size, occasionally becoming as big as a nut, and commonly occur during pregnancy.

(2) Deep type: these can be felt along the main trunks of nerves, for example, the brachial.

(3) Multiple: brown macules, 'café-au-lait' spots, may occur without any tumours. But they may also occur in association with (a) tumours in the skin, or (b) enormous, pendulous, pigmented tumours, or very widespread pigmented lesions covering the bathing-suit area. These macules are found in 90 per cent of cases of neuro-fibromatosis.

Central nervous system abnormalities and bony changes also occur.

DIAGNOSIS

This is made by the café-au-lait spots and the pedunculation of the lesions.

TREATMENT

Excision when required.

Lipoma

These are soft rounded swellings occurring in the dermis and/or subcutaneous tissue, singly or severally, and as their name suggests, they are composed of fat cells.

They are usually found on the shoulders and back, and sometimes cause discomfort to their owner when supine.

Very rarely they become malignant.

TREATMENT

is by excision.

Chondrodermatitis helicis

This is a chronic inflammatory nodular lesion formed on the rim of the ear. Trauma undoubtedly predisposes, and males predominate.

PATHOLOGY

There is hyperkeratosis and acanthosis, with a mild dermal infiltrate. Cystic degeneration of the cartilage may occur.

CLINICAL FEATURES

The onset is sudden, with the appearance of a hard round painful nodule, of reddish colour, often covered with a small crust. The principal symptom is disturbance of sleep through lying on the lesion.

DIAGNOSIS

This is made from solar keratosis, and squamous cell carcinoma, none of which causes acute pain on pressure.

TREATMENT

Excision, or curettage followed by gentle cauterization.

Solar Keratosis

The condition occurs as a rough horny lesion, on areas exposed to strong sunlight, usually in fair-skinned individuals, any time after the age of about 40. Malignant change occurs in a small minority of cases, the developing squamous cell carcinoma being very slow growing, and with little tendency to metastasize. Such a change is only likely several years after the onset of the lesion.

PATHOLOGY

Hyperkeratosis, acanthosis, papillomatosis and a chronic inflammatory infiltrate in the dermis can be seen.

Evidence of malignant change must be excluded.

CLINICAL FEATURES

The lesions are papular, and vary in size from a pin-head to a coin (Fig. 59). The shape is variable, and the outline well defined. The surface is rough and horny, and when removed bleeding occurs. Sometimes the scale is heaped up in a lump, at other times it is thin and wafer-like; in both instances it is quite adherent. The colour of the lesion is brownish. When there is inflammation or induration around the edge, malignant change must be considered.

DIAGNOSIS

The condition must be distinguished from senile warts, which are soft and not covered with a scale.

TREATMENT

Cauterization, superficially applied, is usually quite sufficient for a good result. 5–10 per cent salicylic acid in collodion, but 5 per cent 5-fluorouracil ointment applied daily for 2–3 weeks is more effective, though causing some discomfort during this time. At the end of the period, the daily application of a steroid cream will soon dispel it.

Granuloma Pyogenicum (Granuloma telangiectaticum)

This occurs as a single, soft, raspberry-like tumour, at any age, in either sex. The cause is unknown, but it is often preceded by minor trauma, such as a penetration of the skin by a thorn.

PATHOLOGY

The epidermis is very thin, because of the great number of newly formed and dilated capillaries which press up against the epidermis, flattening it.

CLINICAL FEATURES

The onset is sudden. The lesion is nodular, and pea to cherry size (Fig. 60). The surface is smooth and glistening, although some areas

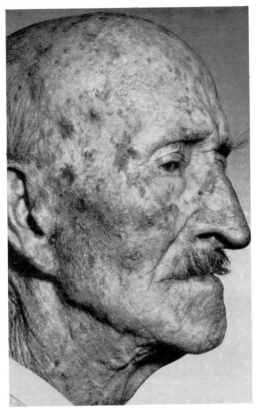

FIG. 59. Solar keratoses (Dr E. Waddington).

may be slightly ulcerated. It looks like an over-ripe fruit. The colour is bright red (Plate 34), due to the excess of capillaries within. Sites commonly affected are the finger, hand, leg, or back. The lesion bleeds easily, and may alarm the patient.

DIAGNOSIS

This is made by the rapid onset, and the tendency to bleeding.

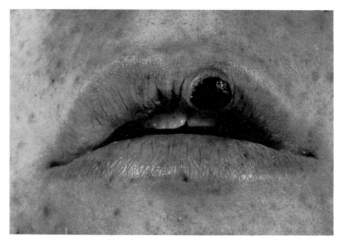

Fig. 60. Granuloma pyogenicum (Institute of Dermatology, University of London).

TREATMENT

Excision followed by cauterization of bleeding surfaces.

PROGNOSIS

The tumour may recur, however skilful the operation.

Kerato-Acanthoma

Molluscum Sebaceum

This term describes a cherry-sized, shell-like tumour, which usually occurs in adults, and in males more often than females. It undergoes spontaneous involution within several months, leaving a depressed and atrophic scar. The cause is unknown.

PATHOLOGY

The microscopical appearance is so like that of a low-grade squamous-cell carcinoma, that differentiation is often impossible.

In this condition, however, the cell changes of carcinoma are absent, and there is a very limited degree of invasiveness.

CLINICAL FEATURES

The onset is quite rapid, and full size is attained in a few weeks. The lesion is round and firm, with a central crater containing horny material (Plate 35). The lesion may grow to a size of 2 or 3 inches, remains well demarcated, and seems to be stuck on the skin. It is flesh-coloured. Commonest sites are the face, backs of the hands and forearms.

TREATMENT

Curettage followed by cauterization is best.

Leucoplakia

This is simply a hyperkeratosis occurring on a mucous membrane (Fig. 61) and is discussed on page 211.

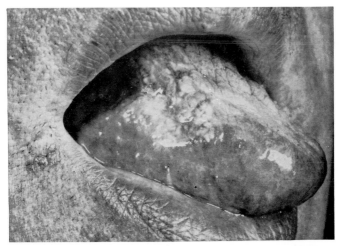

FIG. 61. Leucoplakia. Sharply defined irregular white patches (Institute of Dermatology, University of London).

MALIGNANT TUMOURS

Basal Cell Carcinoma

Rodent ulcer, or basal cell epithelioma

The condition to be described is best known by the three names above. None of them is absolutely correct. Although most of these tumours arise from basal cells, some few do not. Rodent ulcer is the oldest of the synonyms, but many of these tumours do not ulcerate. An epithelioma means any tumour derived from the epithelium.

Whichever name is preferred, the lesions are recognized as superficial or deep nodules or indurated ulcers, usually on the face, but sometimes elsewhere. They rarely metastasize, but ulcerate the surrounding tissue in which they lie.

They are uncommon before the age of 40, and males are more prone than females. They are the commonest form of skin cancer accounting for approximately 70 per cent of the total.

PATHOLOGY

The tumour cells are very characteristic. They are large, oval, and stain deep blue-black with haematoxylin. Although they may appear in the epidermis, they commonly lie in various groups in the dermis, the cells inside the group being haphazardly arranged, whilst those all around the edge of the group are arranged as a palisade.

An inflammatory reaction in the dermis varies according to the rate of growth of the tumour, being more pronounced in rapidly growing lesions.

CLINICAL SIGNS

The onset is insidious. The lesion is nodular, growing from pin-head to pea-size, or somewhat larger. The edge is pearly, shiny and raised, and this is a notable characteristic. The surface of the lesion may be unbroken, or ulcerated. When the crust is removed the surface bleeds easily. Commonest sites are the face (Figs. 62, 63) and forehead (Fig. 64), but the scalp (Fig. 65), forearms, or trunk (Fig. 66) may become involved.

There are three common clinical types of lesion. 1. Button-like,

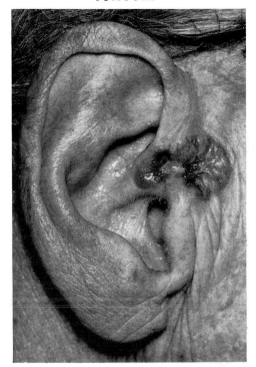

Fig. 62. Basal cell carcinoma (Department of Dermatology, Addenbrooke's Hospital).

or nodulo-ulcerative. 2. Pigmented nodulo-ulcerative. 3. Fibrotic type, appearing as a slightly raised, firm, yellowish plaque, which usually ulcerates.

DIAGNOSIS

This is made by the long history of slow growth, and the appearance of the pearly-edged nodule. A biopsy will, of course, clinch the diagnosis.

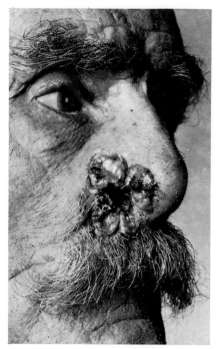

FIG. 63. Basal cell carcinoma in advanced stage (Dr E. Waddington).

A rapid method of confirming a clinical diagnosis is by cyto-diagnosis, a manoeuvre in which one scrapes the ulcerated area, applies the tissue to a slide, and stains with haematoxylin and eosin. A positive result will show numbers of the cells peculiar to this condition.

DIAGNOSIS

This is made by the long history, slow growth, pearly and waxy edge, and biopsy. Squamous cell carcinoma grows faster, sometimes half an inch in 3 months, and is white and opaque. Kerato-acan-

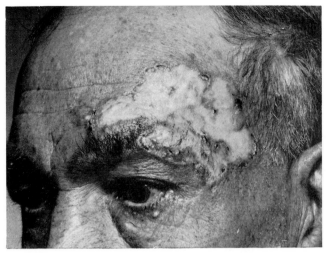

Fig. 64. Basal cell carcinoma, showing a marked rolled edge (Dr E. Waddington).

thoma grows rapidly, stops growing within 4–8 weeks, and does not ulcerate.

TREATMENT
Excision, X-rays; cautery, or diathermy, combined with curettage.

PROGNOSIS
A small percentage recur, however effective the treatment seems to have been.

Squamous Cell Carcinoma

This differs greatly from the basal cell carcinoma, being a true invasive tumour, which develops in normal tissue, or in a pre-existing lesion, such as leucoplakia, or as a sequal to a senile keratosis. It occurs more commonly in elderly people.

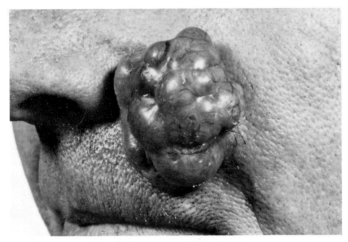

Fig. 65. Cystic basal cell carcinoma.

PATHOLOGY

Masses of irregularly grouped epithelial cells teem downwards to invade the dermis. These masses contain flat prickle cells very distorted in size and shape, intercellular fibrils, and, dotted about, shiny horny pearls. In reality, these 'pearls' are composed of concentrically arranged layers of horn cells enclosing a central area of keratinization, or horn.

In rapidly growing lesions there are many atypical cells, as well as mitoses. The degree of malignancy can be estimated by consideration of the ratio of the differentiated to undifferentiated cells.

CLINICAL FEATURES

The onset is gradual. The lesions may begin as hard nodules, sometimes with a warty surface; or as flat scaly indurated lesions. When the growth is 1 or 2 cm in diameter, ulceration occurs, and the edge of the ulcer becomes thick and everted. The surface may be papillomatous, or like a cauliflower, and have a very smelly exudate.

Occasionally, the lesions do not ulcerate. Localized lymphadenitis may be present, and metastases should be sought.

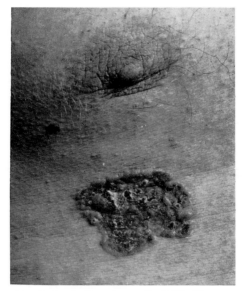

FIG. 66. Basal cell carcinoma (Dr E. Waddington).

Ulcerative lesions fluoresce orange under Wood's light (see p. 133).

DIAGNOSIS

This is made by the comparatively rapid growth, the marked induration, and biopsy, or cytodiagnosis.

TREATMENT

Excision is the best method for most lesions. X-rays give good results for lesions under an inch in diameter. The patient must be regularly examined for 5 years, as if a relapse occurs, it is most often between 2 and 3 years later. When metastasis to regional nodes is present, it should be treated by a combination of X-rays and bleomycin. Bleomycin is a glycopeptide antibiotic obtained from streptomyces verticillus.

Paget's Disease of the Nipple

Carcinoma of the Nipple

This is a rare tumour, which involves the female nipple or areola, and is nearly always unilateral. Occasionally, it affects males. It normally occurs between the ages of 40 and 60. It is sometimes confused with eczema. It is part of a 'field change' in which there is almost invariably underlying carcinoma of the breast.

PATHOLOGY
Paget cells are large, and easily visible in the epidermis. Around them is a clear space. Their nuclei are large, round and pale. Early lesions often fail to show Paget cells. There is also a marked inflammatory infiltrate.

CLINICAL FEATURES
The onset is insidious. The early lesion is papular, and round and well defined. At first small, it enlarges up to palm size. It is red and the surface is scaly, which when removed reveals red, eroded or oozing surfaces. In this state it is very like eczema.

The lesion gradually becomes indurated, infiltrated and sometimes ulcerated. The nipple may become retracted or destroyed (Plate 36).

Untreated, the lesion is relentlessly progressive, and lymph node enlargement and metastases are common in advanced cases.

DIAGNOSIS
This is made by its unilateral distribution, its induration and chronicity, and failure to respond to simple remedies.

It must be distinguished from *eczema* of the nipple, which is normally bilateral and in which the lesion is soft and responds to simple measures.

TREATMENT
There is a matter of some controversy and generally depends on the staging of the tumour, a subject dealt with in surgical textbooks.

Radical mastectomy, and removal of axillary lymph nodes,

followed by X-rays, is the method of choice of many, in advanced disease.

EXTRA-MAMMARY PAGET'S DISEASE

This is found on the vulva and peri-anal areas. The mammary gland is a modified sweat gland, and extra-mammary lesions are considered to be intra-epidermal metastases from an apocrine gland carcinoma. Systemic metastases are rare.

Mycosis Fungoides

This is an uncommon, chronic and invariably fatal disease, which is accompanied and preceded by severe itching. It only affects adults, and rarely females. The cause is unknown.

The name is misleading as it has nothing to do with fungus infection, but is a form of reticulosis.

CLINICAL FEATURES

There are 3 clear-cut stages:

1. Eczematous, which lasts a few months or years.
2. Infiltrative plaque, often accompanied by exfoliative derma-titis. In this stage death may occur, or the disease may continue into the third stage.
3. Tumour; these infiltrated thick lesions break down to form deep sloughing ulcers. Death follows from exhaustion within a few months or years.

Duration

Death occurs within 5 years of the onset, unless treatment is given.

TREATMENT

This varies with the stage of the disease. First stage: topical or intralesional steroids, ultra-violet radiation, or psoralens combined with UVA (PUVA p. 66). Second stage: superficial X-rays, metho-trexate, cleomycin, U.V.R. or PUVA. Third stage: radiation with electron beams, steroids and/or methotrexate, or cleomycin.

In the first and second stages, all these treatments cause remission of the disease, particularly PUVA.

Malignant Melanoma

This rare tumour arises from a pigmented naevus (p. 260), or apparently normal skin, and is characterized by a blue-black nodule which gradually increases in size.

It occurs at any age although rare before puberty, and is more frequent in women.

PATHOLOGY

The malignant changes almost always occur at the epidermo-dermal junction. The naevus cells already there, as part of a pigmented naevus, suddenly become bloated, and take in more melanin, so that they stain very darkly. The cell nuclei also enlarge, and mitosis is seen. Soon the cells proliferate and flood into the dermis and epidermis, and evidence of a breakthrough into the lymphatics and blood vessels may be noted.

CLINICAL FEATURES

The onset is insidious, or quite rapid. The lesion may present as a nodule, a flat superficial patch, or develop from a solar lentigo on actinic-damaged skin. The colour is most striking being blue-black, or jet black, which the patient will comment on, and at the edge of the lesion a red halo may be seen. The sites commonly affected are the head and neck (Fig. 67), and then the lower extremities, but no area is exempt, a melanotic whitlow being one of the more unusual sites. Lymphadenopathy occurs early, and melanuria, melanaemia, and wasting soon follow.

Its course is unpredictable.

DIAGNOSIS

This is made by the sudden increase in size and depth of colour of a pigmented naevus, and by bleeding and ulceration of the lesion.

When the tumour arises from normal skin, a small black or brown spot appears followed by rapid growth.

The diagnosis must be made from dark haemangiomas, traumatic blood blisters and pigmented basal-cell carcinomas.

TREATMENT

These lesions must be treated as emergencies, and any suspected

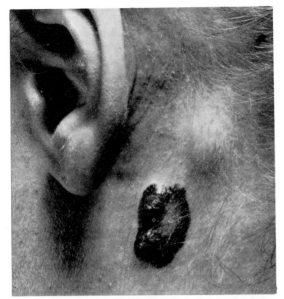

FIG. 67. Melanoma (Institute of Dermatology, University of London).

lesion should be widely and deeply excised and subjected to biopsy, with immediate frozen sections. A simple incisional biopsy is fraught with the danger of causing prompt metastases.

Associated lymph nodes are treated by block dissection, or endo-lymphatic therapy, by injection with isotopes.

PROGNOSIS
This depends on the degree of dermal infiltration. Mortality in-creases with age.

Hodgkin's Disease

This is a systemic disease of the lymphoid-reticular system affecting primarily and predominantly lymph nodes. In a few cases, the skin may be first affected

CLINICAL FEATURES

In most cases there is generalized itching. Urticarial, bullous, vesicular or papular eruptions occur. Alopecia and purpuric lesions may also appear, and herpes zoster as a complication should not be forgotten. Splenomegaly and pyrexia are also present.

TREATMENT

X-rays cause disappearance of the lesions which tend to recur. Numerous and complicated cytotoxic regimes are now in force for the systemic manifestations. These also help skin lesions. Splenectomy helps in some cases.

Leukaemia

Involvement of the skin in the lymphatic and myeloid forms is very similar, but is most common in the lymphatic form.

In the *chronic* leukaemias, nodules and tumours are common. In the *acute* leukaemias, purpuric, haemorrhagic bullous and ulcerative lesions are more usual.

Herpes zoster and exfoliative dermatitis (as in Hodgkin's disease) should not be forgotten as possible complications of the disease.

TREATMENT

Immunosuppressants, steroids or chlorambucil are used.

Metastatic Carcinoma

Cancer of the skin, secondary to a primary source in the body, is very rare. Cancer of the breast is the commonest form to metastasize in this way. Skin metastases have been seen with hypernephromas, gastric, lung and uterine cancers.

Skin Changes related to Internal Cancer

Itching may be generalized in Hodgkin's disease, lymphatic leukaemia, cancer of the breast, stomach, pancreas, lungs or prostate.

Urticaria may also occur with the above-mentioned conditions.

Flushing of the face, and upper part of the body, may occur with carcinoid tumours.

CHAPTER 20

Congenital and Hereditary Diseases

Ichthyosis: Palmar and Solar Keratosis: Haemangiomas:
Lentigo: Naevus Flammeus: Cellular Naevi: Warty Naevi

Introduction

Congenital diseases can be evident at or before birth or be manifest later. They may or may not be inherited; and not all inherited disorders are congenital. Fortunately, the great majority of congenital skin diseases are rare, and many of them are collector's pieces; the minority are more common, and some of them will be described here.

For a description of the factors responsible for the appearance of congenital affections, specialized text-books should be consulted. Unlike the majority of disorders with which the dermatologist has to deal, the question of treatment of congenital skin diseases in the case of most disorders is overshadowed by the knowledge that much improvement is difficult to obtain, and in some of the more serious and rare conditions, life can only be precariously enjoyed.

The problem of classification is difficult because the clinician prefers the use of terms which describe the tissue affected by the disease, whilst the geneticist requires his own special terminology, dependent upon the transmitting factors of the disease.

Ichthyosis

This common condition is characterized by a dry, rough, and scaly skin (Fig. 68), sometimes resembling fish-scales (*ichthus*—a fish), which most severely affects the extensor surfaces, and usually spares the flexor ones.

All degrees of the condition may be seen, from that of an infant

Ectodermal Disorders	Mesodermal Disorders	Ecto- and Meso-dermal Disorders
*Ichthyosis	*Epidermolysis bullosa (simple and dystrophic types)	*Neurofibromatosis
Congenital ichthyosiform erythroderma		
*Keratosis of palms and soles		Acanthosis nigricans (juvenile type)
*Congenital alopecia		
*Albinism White forelock	Congenital lymphoedema	
Pachonychia congenita	Urticaria pigmentosa	
	*Naevus flammeus	
Congenital absence of nails	*Simple haemangioma	
Congenital antidrotic ectodermal defect Porphyria	*Cavernous haemangioma Blue naevus	

N.B. Only those marked with an asterisk are described in this book.

encased in a bone-dry suit of 'scale armour', to a skin whose perfection is marred by slight scaling. This latter form is extremely common. It is called ichthyosis vulgaris, and is dominantly inherited. Other varieties are classified according to their inheritance.

CAUSE

Inheritance
A relevant history can nearly always be obtained.

Age
The common variety is seen between the ages of 1 and 4, and is unusual in early infancy.

Sex
Males are slightly more affected than females.

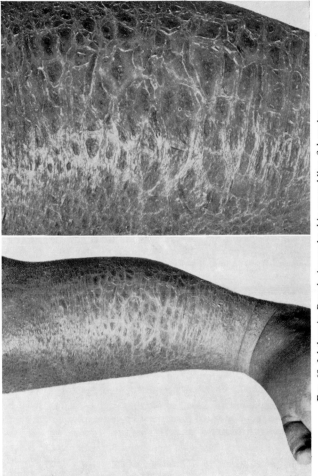

FIG. 68. Ichthyosis. Rough dry scaly skin resembling fish-scales.

PATHOLOGY

Hyperkeratosis is present, which accounts for the thickening of the skin with a reduction or complete absence of the granular layer. The sweat glands are usually normal, but the sebaceous glands may be absent, or atrophic.

CLINICAL FEATURES

There are no lesions, as such. Dry scaling, and thickening of the skin on the extensor surfaces predominates. The scales are centrally fixed to the skin, and are loose and slightly turned up at the edges. The tops of hair-follicles may be capped by hard keratotic papules.

The hair is thin and dry. The amount of scaling and hair and nail involvement depends on the severity of the affection.

Many patients show one or more signs of atopy (p. 39).

TREATMENT

Irritants, such as detergents and soaps, must be avoided. Greasy applications, such as oily cream B.P.C., E.45 cream, or a mixture of 3 parts olive oil to 1 part of glycerine are helpful. Bran or Oilatum oil (Stiefel) in a bath are soothing. Carbamide (urea) 10 per cent in an emulsifying cream (Calmurid) is a useful application, twice daily, after washing or bathing. Steroid preparations are not merited for this condition.

A warm sunny climate is better than a cold one.

Keratosis of Palms and Soles

Tylosis

This condition is characterized by symmetrical thickening of the skin of the palms and soles, of varying degrees. Apart from being congenital, it is also often hereditary. In some ways it appears to be related to ichthyosis.

Haemangiomas

These naevoid lesions are composed of newly formed blood vessels, and are present at birth, or appear within the first few months of life. They are very common, and there are three main types:

1. Simple haemangioma.
2. Cavernous haemangioma.
3. Naevus flammeus (flat haemangioma, or port-wine stain).

Simple Haemangioma

This is a bright red raised soft tumour, often appearing like a strawberry (Fig. 69). About 10 per cent of infants have them and they are found more commonly in girls.

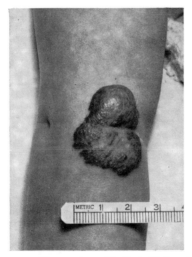

FIG. 69. Haemangioma (Dr G. A. Hodgson).

PATHOLOGY

This shows an increase and dilatation of capillaries.

CLINICAL FEATURES

The lesions vary in size, up to a medium-sized strawberry. They occur anywhere, and are generally single.

TREATMENT

None is usually required, as they involute spontaneously by the age of five years, leaving a better end result than operative measures can accomplish. Treatment is only indicated where the lesion interferes with sight or sucking.

Cavernous Haemangioma

These lesions are composed of fully mature blood vessels. They are far more solid to palpation than the simple variety, but scarcely fade on pressure. They appear shortly after birth and usually disappear by the age of 5 or 6.

Naevus Flammeus

This is characterized by one or several dark-red or pink patches, irregular in outline (Plate 37), and not raised above the skin.

It is formed by a diffuse telangiectasia of mature blood vessels in the dermis.

CLINICAL FEATURES

The lesions are usually unilateral on the face or neck (Fig. 70), but other areas may be affected. Lesions can be of any size and may involve mucous membranes. Crying, coughing, or exposure to cold alters the lesions' colour.

TREATMENT

None is really satisfactory, and if plastic surgery is to be used, it should be used as soon as possible. Cosmetic creams can be used to hide the blemish, which is usually a great psychological handicap to the individual.

Lentigo

A small brown circular macule, due to an increased number of melanocytes at the dermo-epidermal junction.

CLINICAL FEATURES

They normally appear in childhood. They may increase in pregnancy and Addison's disease.

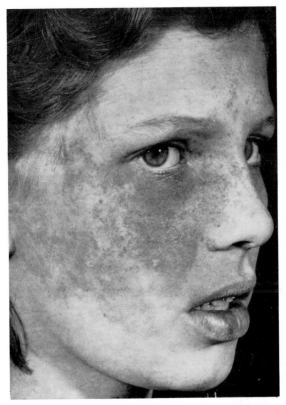

FIG. 70. Naevus flammeus (Institute of Dermatology, University of London).

DIAGNOSIS

From freckles by their darker colour and scattered distribution, and the fact that they do not darken in colour, or multiply on exposure to sun. Seborrhoeic keratoses have a granular and slightly keratotic surface.

Naevi

A naevus is a circumscribed developmental defect of the skin. Naevi involve one tissue, which is commonly present in excess, and associated local dysplasia of other tissues is usual. The term *hamartoma* is now often used synonymously with naevus.

Pigmented Naevus

(Melanocytic naevus, cellular naevus, mole)

A pigmented naevus is formed by proliferation of the melanocytes at the dermo-epidermal junction, and is a developmental defect.

Many of the public consider most moles to be dangerous and prone to change into malignant growths: fortunately this is rarely true.

From the histological point of view there are three types of pigmented naevus:

1. *Junctional naevus*
2. *Intradermal naevus*
3. *Compound naevus*

The *junctional naevus* may show (1) active formation of naevus cells at the epidermo-dermal junction only, or (2) activity also in the dermis in nest formation without an inflammatory infiltrate, or scattered simply in the dermis, with an inflammatory infiltrate. In the second instance, the malignancy potential is greater and this problem can only be settled by a pathologist.

The *intradermal naevus* shows cells in the dermis without epidermo-dermal junction activity.

The *compound naevus* shows naevus cells in both areas.

CLINICAL FEATURES

The *junction type* of naevus appear at birth or any time afterwards. It is a macule or papule, brown or smooth, and hairless. It may occur anywhere on the skin or muco-cutaneous surfaces.

The *intradermal type* is a papule, usually hairy, well defined, smooth, flesh coloured or brown. It is most common on the face and neck.

The *compound type* vary from a slightly raised plaque to mammilated nodule. They are usually very dark in colour.

DIAGNOSIS

In children, this has to be made from vascular naevi which are rather reddish than brown, and the colour may be expelled by pressure.

In adults, the *seborrhoeic keratosis* has a dull granular surface, which is yellowish brown. A *pigmented basal cell carcinoma* shows dilated vessels on the surface, and there is a history of slow growth. A *fibroma* is a firm dermal nodule.

TREATMENT

Excision and routine biopsy is the best treatment for pigmented naevi. The great majority of them are harmless (see p. 250).

Warty Naevus

These lesions may be single or multiple, and are brown in colour.

Naevus cells may be absent or not, depending on the presence of an associated pigmented naevus.

Clinically they appear as hyperpigmented patches, or warty streaks following the course of a nerve, and are then often called linear naevi.

TREATMENT

Cauterization or diathermy. Sometimes surgical excision is required.

Bibliography

The following books are amongst those which have been consulted, and are recommended for further reading.

FREGERT S. (1974) *Manual of Contact Dermatitis*. Year Book Med. Publ.

LEVER W.F. (1975) *Histopathology of the Skin*. Pitman Medical, London.

ROOK A., WILKINSON D.S. & EBLING F.T.G. (1972) *Textbook of Dermatology*. Blackwell Scientific Publications, Oxford and Edinburgh. The most comprehensive book of all, but too large for the undergraduate.

TURK J.L. (1974) *Immunology in Clinical Medicine*. Heinemann, London.

WILKINSON D.S. (1973) *The Nursing and Management of Skin Diseases*. Faber & Faber, Lonndon.

British National Formulary 1976–78.

Examination Questions

Samples of multiple choice questions set in recent examinations for the Final M.B.

1. Generalized itching can be a symptom of:
   (a) gout; (b) lymphatic leukaemia; (c) drug reactions; (d) Hodgkin's disease; (e) chronic renal failure.

2. The following conditions may cause erythema nodosum:
   (a) streptococcal infection; (b) sarcoidosis; (c) tuberculosis; (d) syphilis; (e) leprosy.

3. Hyperpigmentation can be well marked in:
   (a) Cushing's syndrome; (b) haemochromatosis; (c) Addison's disease; (d) pregnancy; (e) lichen planus.

4. The buccal mucosa may be affected in:
   (a) lichen planus; (b) Addison's disease; (c) pemphigoid; (d) warts; (e) leprosy.

5. Contraindications to vaccination are:
   (a) Infantile eczema; (b) pregnancy; (c) systemic lupus erythematosus; (d) previous smallpox infection; (e) sarcoidosis.

6. Diffuse alopecia may be found in:
   (a) Psoriasis; (b) systemic lupus erythematosus; (c) hyperthyroidism; (d) hypothyroidism; (e) secondary syphilis; (f) puerperal states.

7. The hands are commonly affected in:
   (a) Contact dermatitis; (b) scabies; (c) basal cell carcinoma; (d) chickenpox; (e) discoid lupus erythematosus.

Approximate Metric and Imperial Equivalents

Weight

1 mg = 0·016 gr   1 gr = 60 mg
1 g = 15 gr   1 dr = 4 g
     = 0·03 oz (avoir, apoth) 1 oz = 30 g
     = 0·25 dr   1 lb = 0·45 kg
1 kg = 2·2 lb

Fluid Measure

1 ml = 15 minim   1 m   = 0·06 ml
      = 0·04 fl oz   1 fl oz = 30 ml
1 litre = 35 fl oz   1 pint = 0·5 litre
      = 1·76 pints   1 gal = 4·5 litre
      = 0·22 gallons

Index